The simple **1:1:1** formula for
fast and sustained weight loss

**1 protein
1 carb
1 fat**
At every
meal

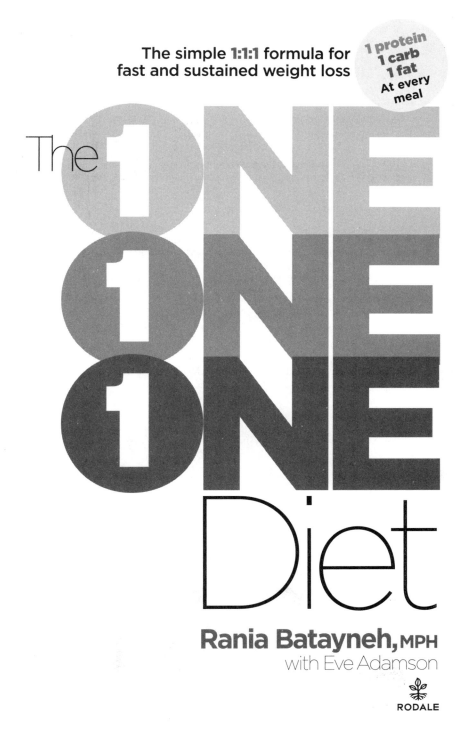

The **1ONE 1ONE 1ONE** Diet

Rania Batayneh, MPH

with Eve Adamson

RODALE

© 2014 by Rania Batayneh, MPH

Rodale books may be purchased for business or promotional use or for special sales. For information, please write to:
Special Markets Department, Rodale, Inc., 733 Third Avenue, New York, NY 10017

Printed in the United States of America
Rodale Inc. makes every effort to use acid-free ♾, recycled paper ♺.

Book design by Chris Rhoads
Cover photography by Beth Bischoff

Library of Congress Cataloging-in-Publication Data is on file with the publisher.
ISBN-13: 978-1-62336-032-0 trade hardcover

Distributed to the trade by Macmillan

2   4   6   8   10   9   7   5   3   1   trade hardcover

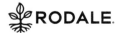

We inspire and enable people to improve their lives and the world around them.
rodalebooks.com

Contents

Acknowledgments

would like to start off by thanking my parents, Afaf and Mohammad, for giving me opportunities that have paved the way for both the scientific and artistic aspects of my career and life. Mom, you taught me how to create and bring beauty to the things that I love doing. I shared your creativity with many of my clients, in the form of recipe ideas as well as inspiring words of motivation—nobody says it better than you. Dad, you showed me the importance of dedicating myself to a career that I love that also helps others, and you gave me a mind to understand the complex technical aspects of health and nutrition.

I would also like to thank my brothers and sisters: Sam, Hilda, and Linda. Your support and encouragement during this journey has meant everything to me.

This book could not have been possible without my son, Amir, my Amouri. I started writing this book when I found out I was pregnant with you and the book's release falls a week after your 2nd birthday. You are woven into every page as I seek to make the world a better, more healthful, more sane place for you. You are the best gift in my life and everything I do is for you.

Thanks to Alex Glass, my literary agent, who always knows the right thing to say.

Thanks to Eve Adamson—what a journey this has been! You understood the concept of *The One One One Diet* from the start. Thank you for the countless hours on the phone and emails back and forth—sometimes I just called or emailed you to say "thank you" for being you, but we both know how much time we spent building and creating together. You were there for me this entire journey, both personally and professionally, and I can't thank you enough for all of your time and dedication! I look forward to the next opportunity to work together.

Thanks to Kate Schlag, an organized and energetic intern from the start. As your pursue your career in nutrition, I hope that I have guided you and given you the tools you need for lifelong success.

Words cannot express my gratitude to my editor, Trisha Calvo, for believing in this project from the beginning, and for her professional advice and assistance in polishing this manuscript. A special thanks also to Ursula Cary, Jess Fromm, Erin Williams, Chris Rhoads, Beth Bischoff, Brent Gallenberger, Aly Mostel, Emily Weber, and the rest of the team at Rodale Books.

Finally, I owe so much to my clients, who have shared their stories with readers in this book, as well as those who, throughout the years, taught me so much about what works and what doesn't. This book is built upon your weight loss successes! Thank you for allowing me to work with you on your journey toward optimal health and wellness.

Introduction

"To eat is a necessity, but to eat intelligently is an art."

—Francois de La Rochefoucauld

've got just one word for you, and it is the secret to lasting weight loss—weight that goes away and stays away for good. The word is just this: one.

Say it three times: one, one, one. Now think of it like this: 1:1:1.

To lose weight, gain energy, and look better than you have in years, all you have to do, every time you eat a meal or a snack, is to choose one protein, one carbohydrate, and one fat. Any one you want, but just one of each. Your diet will fall into balance, and so will your body. The end. One protein, one carb, one fat.

But wait! That's not everything! The 1:1:1 approach yields many gifts—as long as you understand how to use it. Although this book is called *The One One One Diet*, my plan absolutely does not fit the criteria of what most people think of as a diet. With 1:1:1, there are no forbidden foods. I'm not kidding! There is no counting anything—not calories, not grams of fiber, not protein grams, nothing. With 1:1:1 you can eat all the foods you love, and still lose weight—and at a rate you might not have experienced before.

Diets aren't the answer. *Balance* is the answer. Balance is what it's all about. Is there really anything wrong with the occasional thick, juicy steak or slice of cheesecake or pile of cheesy nachos? Of course not. Food is fuel, but food can also be fun, pleasurable, even decadent. Why shouldn't you get to enjoy it like all those thin people you know? The truth is that it's not so much about *what* you eat. It's more about *how* you eat, but for some reason, how to eat "normally" eludes most of us.

Sometimes I'm astounded by the misinformation I hear from my clients—the things they believe, the questions they ask, the diet rules they follow. Like:

"A banana isn't a fruit because it's bad for you."

What?

"I ate low-carb all day so I can eat cookies tonight."

Wait, no!

"I could lose weight if I just stopped snacking."

Sigh.

Why is weight loss so hard? My theory is it's because we've deluded ourselves for too long. We believe every new diet plan is the answer to our weight problems. We hop from one diet to another, going all-in at first, then totally throwing in the towel when it doesn't work out. In between dieting, we eat huge amounts of junk that passes for food. We don't take care of ourselves, but most importantly, we eat, move, and live out of balance. We can't find our metaphorical footing, and that's made a lot of people overweight.

There is so much conflicting nutritional information out there that people obviously don't know what they are really supposed to do anymore. Eating didn't used to be so complicated, but people genuinely ask me: "What are humans supposed to eat?" We've lost our natural instincts, and we've lost touch with what our bodies need. We've even lost touch with our own taste preferences. I've asked clients, "What kind of food do you like to eat?"

I get blank stares. They don't even remember.

And don't get me started on nutritionists. Sometimes I think they're all crazy, too. They're all about "Don't eat this" and "Always eat that" and "You have to eat this, not that." Rules, rules, rules. I don't know about you, but I'm a nutritionist and I'm sick of rules—especially the ones that tell me I can't have what I like to eat. Personally, I enjoy a good dessert now and then. I prefer white pasta to whole wheat pasta. Sometimes, I want steak for dinner. Why would I stick to a diet that didn't allow me to eat the foods I like, and required I eat foods I don't like? Especially when the rules aren't even effective! If all that restriction worked, would we have such high rates of obesity in this country? I don't think so.

Still, some people like rules. They beg for rules. My clients often ask me to just write them up a list of rules, or allowed foods. We buy diet books written by celebrities and slavishly follow them—for awhile. Inevitably we rebel against the rules and eat junk anyway. Rules are great until they contradict what we want to do.

We've been living with a lot of nutritional rules in America. They come and go, like fads. First we're supposed to eat low-fat. No, wait, it's low-carb. No, no, none of that matters, it's low-calorie! We're supposed to eat more whole grains, or fewer, or no grains at all. We're supposed to shun white food and eat multicolored food—but only if it's not artificially colored. We're supposed to eat more fruit, or less fruit, or just less sugar all around. We're supposed to eat more vegetables. That will solve everything! Or less red meat, or no meat at all—or only meat and nothing else.

Huh?

Obviously, we're confused. The rules aren't working because of the very fact that they are rules—restrictive rules, elimination rules. Rules are no fun the second you want something you can't have, and then you feel guilty if you break the rules, and then you end up eating things you didn't even really want to eat, just to break the rules out of rebellion—and then you follow them again, out of penance.

It's a mess. We've gotten so far from a realistic idea of what we are supposed to be eating for good health that most of my clients cling desperately to the rules they've heard—at least in theory. Recently, one of my clients told me, "I know how I should be eating."

"That's good!" I said. "And when was the last time you ate the way you know you should be eating?"

"About 6 months ago," she confessed.

If you know how you should be eating, why wouldn't you eat that way? I think it's because of that word *should*.

I had another client tell me, "I'm trying to go low-carb."

"You're *trying* to go low-carb?" I asked. "Why are you just trying? Either you do it or you don't."

"It's hard," she said.

"Then don't do it," I said. "It's hard because it's out of balance."

"But I want to do it," she said.

"Then why just try? Why would you decide to do something, then cheat on yourself?"

If you have to try that hard and it's not working, you aren't on the right plan for you.

Then I have those clients who are always trying to work the system. I had one woman who was previously on Weight Watchers tell me with glee how she's learned to manipulate the points so she can cheat "legally" and eat candy every day.

"Aren't you just cheating yourself?" I asked her.

"I never thought of that," she said. "I thought I was cheating *them*."

Sometimes I throw up my hands at the rules I hear, or the way people interpret them, but the truth is that we're all just being human. There's nothing wrong with *you*. I believe what's wrong are the rules. To eat better, to lose weight, to feel better, to get healthier, you don't need a rulebook.

You need a strategy.

About Me and My Strategy

My name is Rania Batayneh (it's pronounced ba-TIE-nuh), and I'm a nutritionist with a master's degree in public health (MPH). I'm also the daughter of an endocrinologist and an interior designer, so I grew up in a household that valued science over hype but that also valued beauty and pleasure. I learned a rational perspective from my father, and an artistic one, as well as a passion for cooking, from my mother. This fusion of art and science helped me to develop my unique perspective on balance. I've counseled and guided thousands of clients toward the better health and weight loss they never thought they could accomplish. I've had an established practice in San Francisco since 2001, called Essential Nutrition for You. I'm also a wellness coach, and people call me America's Eating Strategist because the method I teach my clients works in the real world, for anyone. I am not Hollywood's Eating Strategist. I am not holed up in some movie studio advising famous people about their wheatgrass shots and coffee enemas. I work with regular people every day—people just like you, who work hard and clip coupons and buy things on sale and shop at grocery stores, not necessarily health food stores. I work with people who lead busy professional lives, who might travel three to four times a month, who might still be in school, who might be dating or are married. Some are divorced and finding themselves once again. Many have children. All of them just want to get "losing weight" off their to-do lists.

The people who come to me for help are overweight and aren't sure why or know why but can't break out of their bad eating habits. Some want to lose 10 pounds, and some have more than 200 pounds to lose. My clients eat the food they can afford, the food that's readily available, that they see advertised on television, and that their friends eat. They don't always have much time to eat breakfast at home and pack their snacks, let alone cook anything complicated, but they can't necessarily afford to go out to a restaurant every night (and if they did, what would be okay to order? They aren't sure!).

But my clients would also really like to lose some weight and have more energy. They would like to feel secure about what they're eating, so they don't have to keep worrying about it. They don't want to follow another diet, necessarily, but they want to be slimmer and fitter than they are right now. They come to me for knowledge. They just want *something* to work. They're just like you, and I created 1:1:1 for them. And it works! Over the years, my clients have collectively lost thousands of pounds. (You'll meet some of them in this book.)

I remember the day I first thought of codifying my nutritional strategy with 1:1:1. It was about 7 years ago, and I was on the phone with a client. Back then, I usually met with clients in person, in my office, where I could sit down and examine their food logs and mark them up and show them where they were going out of balance. I've always been about balance, and I've always thought it was silly—not to mention nutritionally unwise—to eliminate whole food groups or convince yourself you can't eat X, Y, or Z, because it will supposedly make you fat. I have always shown my clients how to incorporate all the food groups and all the foods they love into a balanced plan.

With this particular client, however, I didn't have her food log. She had read about me online and contacted me to see how we could work together. I told her that she had to keep a food log. She said that keeping a food log just made her obsess more. She was already using an online food tracker and was devastated when she ate more than 1,000 calories per day. She wanted to know what to do *right now* to lose weight, so I was trying to consider all these factors while explaining to her what she should be eating.

I asked her to describe her typical day of eating for me. When she told me, it was clear to me that she was eating out of balance. However, without the usual benefit of my pen and paper, where I can make pictures and cross things out and tally the protein, carb and fat servings and show people visually what I am talking about, I was having a hard time getting through to her. I had to find an easy formula to explain how she could eat for more effective weight loss. I told her how her choices and pairings weren't working for her, and how she could shift things around during the day to feel better and drop pounds.

I consider myself an articulate person, but for some reason this woman just wasn't getting it. The message wasn't coming through. She couldn't seem to swallow the notion that she could eat fruit and bread and even cookies, but that she had to balance them with foods in other food groups. She kept saying things like, "So, I can have a cookie if I skip the steak, right?" We just weren't communicating.

Then, suddenly, it hit me.

"Let me put it this way," I said. "Every time you eat, have one protein, one carb, one fat."

There was a long pause. Then, she said: "Ohhhhhhh." Suddenly, we were on the same page.

I've used this strategy ever since, with clients who come into my office as well as those I counsel over the phone. Everyone gets it. They still have questions. They still need a food log analysis. They still want to know how to apply 1:1:1 to a lot of different situations. The concept, however, is clear: Balance at every meal and snack will put you back on the right track to eating normally and easing your body back to its natural healthy weight. Yes, 1:1:1 puts *you* back in charge of your diet, so you never have to rely on anyone else to tell you what to eat again.

The simple fact is that diet rules usually don't work. Sure, some people have lost weight using rules, but more often than not, they go off their diets and the pounds come back—and they've brought a few of their friends. That's why this is my mission: to show you why those rules don't work, and to arm you with a strategy that *does* work.

Because, so far, we're not doing very well. According to the National Institutes of Health, among American adults ages 20 years and older, 211.9 million are overweight or obese (and that was in 2009–2010—it may be even higher right now). We don't know what to do, or we think we know but we can't make ourselves do it, or we just give up and don't care anymore and resign ourselves to feeling like less and looking like more than we really are.

I want you to feel like you have more to offer the world. I want you to feel strong and powerful and in charge of your own life. I want you to feel balanced, and when you achieve that, your body will reflect what you feel inside. You will be a more confident manager of your own health and wellness.

I want you to stop punishing yourself. Excess weight is punishment enough for the crazy diet ideas so many people try to follow. I recently read about a celebrity who is coming out with a new line of baked goods full of protein powder and artificial sweeteners. Fake brownie, anyone? If you want to eat a brownie and be healthy, it's not an impossible scenario. Why do you have to eat a disgusting brownie filled with protein powder and weird sweeteners? Talk about punishment! Why can't you just eat a normal brownie and feel fine about it?

You can, people. *You can.*

A strategy is a way to eat the foods you want to eat without prohibitions or punishment. A strategy is about behaviors you can implement daily and consistently for long-term success, without feeling deprived. A strategy isn't something you "go on" and "go off." It's not a rule. A strategy sets you free to live your life the way you want to live it. This is what I'm giving you with 1:1:1.

I'm truly excited about 1:1:1. I think it could help cure America's obesity problem. I want to tell everyone about 1:1:1! I'm often quoted in the media as a nutrition expert and I try to get the message of balance out there as much as I can, but I found that it wasn't enough. Quotes in a magazine or on a popular website might plant a seed, but they don't include any follow-up or detailed explanation of how to implement the strategy.

This is exactly how the book came about. Because I can't bring every single person struggling with weight issues into my office, I want to give you my strategy for healthy eating that will help you lose weight starting right now, and then I want to help you learn how to use it until you know *exactly* what to do. I want to teach you to live without me, or any nutritionist, or any diet book.

I want you to be able to live your life with confidence, feeling good about your dietary choices every day. Forget calories. Forget fat grams. Forget counting carbs. All that counting is *so* 5 minutes ago. You only need to count to one because 1:1:1 is the stuff of normalcy. It's easy, it's real, and it works. I've got the clients to prove it. I'm proof myself! After I had my son, I lost 42 pounds—all the baby weight—in 6 months using the 1:1:1 strategy.

This concept has freed so many people, both women and men, to enjoy their meals again without fear of slowing weight loss or gaining weight. It has also helped hundreds of people come to terms with their love-hate relationship with food. If you can eat anything you want—no food is off-limits, I swear!—but you also understand how to moderate your choices so you never overdo it, you can finally make peace with food.

Now Where Do We Go?

This is America, and this is what we've gotten ourselves into, for many reasons. I'm not going to go into those reasons right now. I'm not here to point any fingers. (Well, maybe a little in Chapter 1!) We've gotten ourselves into a mess, and now it's time to get back out. For now, just know that I'm here to get you back into balance. I want to teach you to eat regular food in a healthy way, to lose weight and feel good, and to do it without a specific meal plan, a "jump start," a cleanse, or any other wacky "solutions" to weight issues. I also want you to be able to eat what you want without having to eliminate any food groups. I want to teach you to strategize. I want to teach you how to eat according to 1:1:1.

Eating according to 1:1:1 sounds simple, and it is, but there are a million ways to make this work in your life, and I'm going to help you find the way to make it work for you. You're going to have questions, and I'm going to answer them. But once you've got it down, you'll understand why it's more than a diet—it's a way of life. You'll re-learn how to eat reasonably, normally, in the way your body expects and requires. You'll restore your body's natural appetite, rhythm, and weight. It's the simplest miracle you'll ever experience.

I'll also take you further. I'll show you how to apply 1:1:1 to your exercise plan (even if you don't have one yet). I'll show you how to use 1:1:1 for more effective stress management. This is truly a comprehensive and life-changing strategy and it can impact and improve everything about your life that is out of balance right now.

I understand where you're coming from. You're tired of everything being so hard. You're tired of eating diet-y food and depriving yourself and feeling guilty about not going to the gym and stressing about your weight, your body, your whole life.

Forget all that. Life doesn't have to be so difficult. I know you just want to live your life and enjoy yourself, but that you also want to be slimmer, trimmer, and healthier. You want to eat like a *normal* person, enjoying the foods you love and not stressing about your jean size. It's not only possible, it's *easy*. You can have it both ways, and 1:1:1 is the key. Are you ready to make it work in *your* life? Then let's get started.

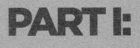

PART I:

Why You Need a Strategy, Not a Diet

CHAPTER ONE

Who Tells You What to Eat—And Why Do You Listen?

Everybody's got an opinion.

I can guarantee that hundreds, even thousands of people are eager to tell you exactly what to eat to lose weight. Your mother-in-law. Your skinny best friend. Your sister. That friend of a friend who just lost 50 pounds. Your doctor, who maybe had a single nutrition class in medical school. The guy sitting next to you on the plane, who just started the Atkins diet, or that vegan girl who works the front desk at your gym and wears T-shirts stating she doesn't eat her friends. Ask "What's the best way to lose weight?" at a party, and the discussion could go on for hours because so many people think they know.

Other sources are more than happy to charge you for the information. The latest issue of your favorite magazine. Diet doctors. Book authors. Diet doctors who are also book authors. Celebrities who know you wish you looked the way they do. Food product manufacturers. Weight loss companies that produce diet meals, ready to ship to your door or your grocery store's freezer case. The diet industry is huge and profitable, even when the economy is down, because no matter how anything else is going in life, everybody wants to be *thin*.

In the world today, a whole lot of people have experience with dieting and weight loss—or have heard about someone else's experience and are happy to pass along the information. If you struggle with your weight, it's amazing how many people are ready to jump in and "help" you.

But there's a big difference between *experience* and *expertise*.

Your neighbor, your trainer, and your mom may have experience losing weight, but they don't have expertise about weight loss or nutrition. They can tell you what they did, but they are *only* telling you what they did. What worked for someone else doesn't necessarily apply to you. You have a completely different body and metabolism, plus different exercise habits and dietary preferences. Maybe you aren't a big fan of meat, or you think a life without cheese sounds barren and depressing, or the idea of weighing yourself at a meeting in front of everybody seems too embarrassing to contemplate. Just remember, when someone tells you about her diet that worked wonders, that's anecdotal. There is a reason anecdotal evidence doesn't count when a drug is being scrutinized by the FDA for approval. It's not an objective measure of what works for everyone.

In fact, studies show all kinds of diets work for certain kinds of people, but they don't work for many others. Some studies have shown that people who are insulin resistant do better on different kinds of diets than people who are insulin sensitive, and others suggest that DNA determines which diet may or may not work for you. A recent study that got a lot of media attention celebrated the Mediterranean diet as the healthiest, not because it was the best diet but because it was the one people were most likely to stick to. And then there's this little interesting study: A company in the United Kingdom wanted to determine whether customized diets were more effective than standard diets. It put 15 people on a weight loss plan that met each individual's preferences, such as wanting cheat days, not wanting to exercise, wanting to cook, etc. They all lost more than 10 pounds in 6 weeks. When the same people were put on a generic diet, only two lost weight, while five gave up and eight people gained weight! From my point of view working with hundreds of people who come to me after diets have failed them, the bottom line is that preference and personalization likely have *everything* to do with sticking to a diet. If you don't stick to your plan, it can't work for you.

Even so, for some reason, people love to copy what other people do. They do it with such hope and optimism. They tell themselves, "I can become *this* now!" or "I'm going to look just like *her!*" or "*He's* my new idol." They convince themselves they can take on somebody else's habits, schedules, tastes, and ways of eating and exercising, even if those things don't fit into their lifestyles. You don't have someone else's body type, or taste, or schedule, or personality, or *life*. You have your very own life, so shouldn't you have your very own way of eating, too?

In my practice, I find that people often have extremely unrealistic expectations about what they can really do over the long term. I think this is why so many diets fail. And even though people know the odds are against them, they really don't believe it. They say they do. "Oh yes, I know, diets don't work, blah blah blah," but deep down, when they hear about a new one, they think that *this time it will be different,* that *this diet* will finally work. They believe that "miracles" have happened for others—celebrities in particular, who are seen as different from the rest of us, like supernatural beings—and that with just the right secrets or tips or tricks, those same miracles (which probably didn't even happen the way they've heard) will happen to them. They begin each new diet passionately, believing that, like a new love interest, *This is the one!*

It's not realistic, but more than that, it's not sustainable. Most people revert back to their old habits and preferences after the thrill of pretending to be somebody else wears off. A week or a month or a few months later, disillusionment sets in. Either the plan was too hard, or it didn't yield the expected results. "But the book said 30 pounds in 30 days!" "But I missed eating bread/cheese/sugar *too much!*" At this point, people tend to go back to eating everything they love and more, as if they were getting revenge on that nasty diet for lying to them. They gain back all the weight they'd lost and lose the good habits they might've picked up. They are through with dieting—that is, until the *next* new diet inspires just as much hope. Maybe *this one* is the answer. Maybe *she* knows what will work for me. Maybe Dr. So-and-So *really gets it.* And the cycle starts all over again.

Here's the problem, as I see it: You are *you.* There are particular reasons why you have gained weight, and there are particular ways that you like to eat, and there are particular ways you can improve your diet. There are weight loss rules that won't work for you, and there are rules that will, but there is absolutely no way to know which is which based on what anybody else tells you. You are completely different than anyone else who ever lost weight on a diet. You are entirely unique.

I think that's pretty cool, actually.

So what will work for you? It might sound strange for me to rail against all these so-called miracle diet books in my own diet book, but here's the difference: Despite what the cover says, *The One One One*

Start-Now Strategy

I'm sure there are plenty of foods you don't want to cut out of your diet, but start thinking about the things you eat out of habit that you don't care that much about. Where could you trim back right now? If you love cheese on your turkey sandwich, have it! But if you snack on unadorned popcorn because you think you should and eat 6 cups of it because it's not satisfying you, replace that with a snack you enjoy more and you could end up eating a lot less.

Diet isn't actually a diet. It's a strategy. It is customizable. It belongs to you. I won't tell you that there are things you cannot eat, because you can eat anything you please. I refuse to tell you that you *have* to eat something, because you don't have to eat anything you don't want to eat. However, I will tell you how to eat, because this is where it's all going to happen for you. And not only will I tell you how to do 1:1:1, but I will tell you how to make 1:1:1 *yours*.

This is a strategy for life. It is something you can do forever because you make it fit you. And that makes all the difference in the world.

However, before I get into the details about exactly how 1:1:1 works and how you can make it work for you, I want to be sure you truly understand why diets and even so-called miracle weight loss secrets are not what they appear to be. I don't want 1:1:1 to be just another diet one-night stand. I want you to truly and fully internalize the notion that there are a lot of people out there telling you what to do, and that none of that matters. You get to decide what makes sense for you and you need to be able to tell the good advice from the bad. I want you to understand when you are being fed hype and PR, and when you are actually being fed true information. I want you to understand at a deep level the difference between experience and expertise. Here are some examples:

• Your best friend calls, excited to tell you that she started drinking her body weight in ounces of water every day and lost 10 pounds. Okay, let's think about this. If she was dehydrated, that could have really helped her. If you're not, it won't do anything for you. You might already drink enough water. If you don't, by all means, drink more water. But water alone is not going to solve your weight issues. Plus, drinking your weight in ounces of water per day could actually harm you. If you weigh 175 pounds right now, it's not healthy to drink 175 ounces of water. That's almost 22 glasses! That might keep you too full to eat much (and cause you to spend most of your day in the bathroom), but you could also dilute the sodium level in your blood too much, which could lead to health problems.

If you drink a lot of soda and you swap it for water, you might lose weight because of the calorie decrease—a 20-ounce regular soda has 240 calories, and that can really add up. But if you don't drink soda, sipping from a water bottle all day long probably won't make the pounds melt off your body. This is what I mean by experience—weight loss was your best friend's *experience*, but that has nothing to do with you. It might work for you. It might not. I just want you to see that it might not.

Food for **Thought**

Are you obsessing about drinking water all day long? Chill out. You probably don't have to force down all that water. If you are sufficiently hydrated, more water is not going to help you lose weight. Most adults need 8 to 12 cups of fluid every day (women are closer to 8 or 9 cups), but it doesn't all have to be water. Soup, tea, coffee, and juice count, too.

Of all the beverage possibilities out there, water is certainly the most healthful. And yes, research shows that water can help some people slim down. In one study, scientists from Virginia Tech recruited 48 overweight men and women aged 55 to 75 who were following a low-calorie diet and asked half of them to drink 2 cups of water before every meal. In 3 months, the water drinkers lost an average of 15.5 pounds, compared to the non-water-drinkers, who lost an average of 11 pounds. However, this is just one small study, and the researchers didn't find a similar effect in younger adults. If you aren't between 55 and 75, overweight, and on a low-calorie diet, it might not apply to you at all. Some people don't digest their food as well if they drink too much water. Instead, choose water over sugary drinks (not only is water calorie free, it quenches your thirst better than sugary beverages) and sip it throughout the day, whenever you think about it. Be sure to drink before, during, and after exercise. Add a slice of fruit to your water to make it taste more interesting, if you want to, and enjoy it.

• Your sister brags about how easy it was for her to lose 15 pounds in a little more than a month. All she had to do was eat more fruits and vegetables. A miracle, right? Eating more of anything to lose weight sounds like a pretty good deal. However, this will not help everyone. If your sister wasn't getting enough nutrients and fiber before, this might have been a great solution for her. Her health probably benefited. She also may have swapped sweets for fruits and replaced other not-so-good-for-you snacks with vegetables—all good from a nutritionist's point of view. However, if you already eat enough fruits and vegetables, increasing your intake isn't likely to help you lose weight. In fact, you might even gain weight because you'll be increasing your calories, assuming you don't change anything else about your diet.

A lot of my clients feel like they have to force themselves to eat more salads and piles of cooked vegetables, even though they don't want to. Vegetables are great and people who don't eat enough of them should certainly try to eat more, but adding them to an already balanced diet isn't necessary, and eating a big salad with dressing and cheese and croutons in addition to your regular meal is like eating two meals. So once again, this was your sister's *experience,* but I want you to gain the expertise to see that it may or may not work for you.

• You read a book by your favorite celebrity, who waxes poetic about how a vegan/gluten-free/all-organic diet is responsible for her healthy, fit physique. Because she is a celebrity and you admire her great body, you might think that whatever she did will certainly have exactly the same effect on you. But you don't know her. For all you know, her diet philosophy could just be part of her "image," cooked up by her public relations staff. Why would you apply that to your personal life? For one thing, you have no proof that she actually did what she says in the book. Maybe she did and maybe she didn't. But even if she did, that was her experience, not yours. You are not her. Maybe she went vegan because she's an animal rights activist, or she quit eating gluten because she has celiac disease. Are you an animal rights activist? If you are, then you might have a really good reason to go vegan, but that doesn't mean it's going to make you look like that celebrity. If you have celiac disease, you should definitely go gluten free, but if you don't have it, a gluten-free diet isn't going to help you lose weight. (I'll talk more about both these issues in the next chapter.) Also consider that this celebrity probably lives a life much different than yours. Do you have the same job? The same family situation? Are you the same age? The same starting weight? Do you exercise the same way she does? Do you have a personal trainer and a personal chef? All these things factor into why something works for one person and not another.

What I want you to understand is that diets may or may not work. If you want to stop experimenting on yourself, then perhaps you should forget all that nonsense. Even if you do have a dietary restriction, you don't necessarily need to go "on a diet." The 1:1:1 strategy is flexible enough to apply to any eating situation or dietary preference. Stick with 1:1:1 and you won't ever be let down by a diet again.

Who Has Expertise?

Now let's talk about someone with expertise. This is quite different than someone with experience. A trained nutritionist or dietitian has expertise. We have learned through extensive and rigorous education how food works in the body. A nutritionist or dietitian may also have experience, but knows that experience is individual and won't use personal experience to guide you. A nutritionist or dietitian knows that expertise is more relevant because it is based on solid research and sound nutritional principles.

A nutritionist or dietitian can tell you why all those diets did or didn't work for all those other people, and why they probably won't work forever. However, even the experts are fallible. A lot of dietitians and nutritionists make a big mistake when they recommend a particular approach: They create meal plans without considering the individual client's lifestyle and preferences. They tell you that you just have to eat certain things in certain amounts if you want to lose weight because that's what has been proven to work. Many believe there is one basic way to eat, whether it's high-fiber, low-fat, or low-carb. They base their plans on a particular segment of scientific research, but without a simultaneous understanding of what will actually help someone stick with a healthy eating plan, the best research in the world is useless.

Who you are, what you like to eat, how you live your life, whether you have children, whether you travel a lot, whether you go on dates, how often you exercise, how often you get hungry—all those things impact your weight. Many nutritionists and dietitians will make lists for you of "allowed" foods and "forbidden" foods. They have rules. They know what *tends* to work for *a lot* of people, but that still doesn't mean it will work for you. Plus the restrictive nature of the diet plans alone are often unsustainable, especially for people who really love to eat or have certain food weaknesses. What if somebody told you that you could never eat sugar again? Or cheese? Or that you could never have another glass of wine? Sure, it makes sense that you shouldn't eat things that have contributed to your excessive weight gain, *in theory*. But that's not how people work.

My approach is different. As a nutritionist and a certified wellness coach with a master's degree in public health, I know the science. I know about nutrition. I know what's healthy for the human body and why. But

Food for **Thought**

I call my company Essential Nutrition for You because I emphasize what is essential—to *you.* Maybe in your life, having a doughnut and a cup of coffee while you read the Sunday newspaper is essential. Maybe a glass of wine after a long day at work is essential. Maybe pizza with the kids on movie night is essential. So what if somebody else thinks you shouldn't be eating some or all of these things? If those parts of your life give you pleasure, you should eat them. It's just a matter of finding balance, so you can have what you enjoy in the context of a healthy diet.

I also know people. I know my clients. I know the best diet in the world isn't going to do any good if you don't follow it.

That's why I want you to learn how to eat "right" *all by yourself.* I want you to have a strategy, and I want you to understand why meal plans and shopping lists and rigid rules *are totally unnecessary for significant, lasting weight loss.* Here's the truth: Your neighbor probably lost weight on a low-carb diet because he stopped eating excessive carbohydrates. Your trainer probably lost weight on a vegan diet because he stopped eating excessive fat and started eating more fiber. Your mom probably lost weight with Weight Watchers because she's the type of person who responds to

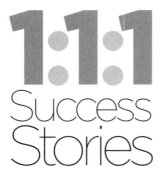

1:1:1 Success Stories

Name: **Mike Gatenby**
Starting weight: **250 pounds**
Current weight: **185 pounds**
Height: **6'0"**

I weighed a healthy 190 pounds when I graduated from college, but over the next several years I slowly gained. By the time I was 29, I was up to 250 pounds and felt awful. I had no energy. My doctor told me my cholesterol was high, my blood sugar was high, and that if I didn't change my diet and lifestyle, I'd be diabetic in 10 years. That was enough to scare the crap out of me and take his advice to make an appointment with Rania.

I wasn't optimistic she could help me, though. I worked long hours and traveled for my job nearly every week. I lived on take-out meals delivered to the office or in restaurants and bars when I was on the road. I spent a lot of time sitting at a desk or on an airplane and didn't have time to exercise. My job was so stressful, I didn't want the added stress of trying to starve myself, and my travel schedule wasn't going to let up any time soon.

being part of a group and loves the support and encouragement she gets from a community. They all lost weight. And they're all at risk for gaining it back if they ever go back to eating the way they did before they began eliminating major food groups or becoming dependent on a program. This is a very real risk for all of them if they didn't incorporate the changes into their lifestyle. If they didn't learn how to eat—if they only went on a diet, and then went off a diet—they are set up to fail.

You, on the other hand, might not lose weight permanently on a low-carb diet or a vegan diet or by going to Weight Watchers, and why put yourself through all that anyway? Wouldn't you rather just learn how to

---

It turned out I was very wrong. Rania taught me that there are strategies you can use when you order take-out or eat at restaurants; that you can put together a healthy meal. As she explained her 1:1:1 approach, I realized I could apply it anywhere. The diet was so sustainable that it didn't feel like a diet at all but more like a new way of life!

One of the best changes I made was to have a morning and afternoon snack. That really kept hunger pangs at bay. I also ate lighter lunches like vegetable soup followed by a turkey sandwich with cheese on whole wheat bread with mustard rather than mayonnaise. I ate more balanced dinners—dodging the bread basket, picking sensible appetizers, and having only one glass of wine. I also started eating more green vegetables and drinking more tomato juice because I can add those things for "free." These are all better nutritional choices than I was making before.

Thanks to Rania's plan, I got down to 185 pounds in 8 months and, in the process, lowered my cholesterol and blood sugar to healthy levels. And the weight has stayed off. I've simply kept on following Rania's advice and stuck with her 1:1:1 eating strategy!

eat normally so you don't even have to think about it? You have to find what will work for you.

What I've Learned from My Clients

I live in a green, tree-filled suburban Portland neighborhood full of small families, with lots of kids running around. I see clients in my home. I invite them in and we sit at my dining room table because the dining room is my favorite room in the house and appropriate for discussing food and nutrition. I give them a glass of water, and we talk. I also "see" a lot of clients over the phone, if they don't live nearby. They call me, and I get to know them. I ask them questions, and they tell me about their lives. I usually learn a lot about exactly who has been advising them about weight loss. I get a lot of interesting information, especially about what *doesn't* work.

Just a few weeks ago, I had a client who came to see me. Her goal was to lose 30 pounds. We sat there in my dining room, and I asked her about her weight loss history.

"I lost 30 pounds 5 years ago," she said. "It was great. I want to do that again."

"How did you do it?" I asked.

"I had a trainer 5 days a week and I was eating low-carb."

"Why did you stop doing that?" I asked. "Did you stop seeing your trainer? Did you get injured? Did you stop eating low-carb?"

"Yes," she said.

This is very telling. She was doing all these things that worked, but obviously they didn't work in the long term. They weren't sustainable. Working out 5 days a week sounds great and ambitious, but what happens when you no longer have the time? Obviously she stopped for some reason.

The same goes for eating low-carb. Many people lose weight in the short term with this approach, but at some point, they get sick of not eating bread or pasta or cake and they go completely in the opposite direction. I actually see this a lot—I have a lot of ex-low-carbers in my practice. Low-carb diets work in the short term, but they're often not sustainable.

I explained to this client that if she wants to lose 30 pounds again, she can do it in a way that will keep it off because it won't be so miserable. She perked right up. Now, she's on her way. She's already lost 6 pounds in 3 weeks.

Another client bragged to me about how she was on Weight Watchers, and was able to eat pizza and Snickers bars while staying within her points. *Another Weight Watchers cheater,* I thought to myself.

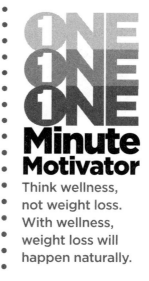

One One One Minute Motivator

Think wellness, not weight loss. With wellness, weight loss will happen naturally.

"If that is working, why are you here?"

"Because I'm not losing weight," she said. "It's not working, but I don't understand it because I'm staying within my points." I realized she just trusted the program to work, no matter how she manipulated it. She thought if she followed the rules, they would work, no matter what. There is nothing wrong with eating the occasional slice of pizza or Snickers bar, but not at the same meal, and not all the time.

"It's not working because it's not balanced," I said. "Points don't guarantee balance."

I'm working right now with another client who used to be a runner. Running helped her keep her weight around 160 pounds, which was a relatively healthy weight for her 5-foot, 9-inch height. Then one day, she broke her foot. Now she weighs 200 pounds.

"What were you doing? Drinking wine every night when your foot was propped up in that cast?"

"Yes," she admitted.

She helped me to see that people don't realize that changing just one thing (in this case, exercise) can make a huge difference in weight, either positively or negatively. Weight is dependent on balance and when you shift that balance, you must account for it somewhere. There is nothing wrong with a glass of wine in the evening if it agrees with you and you enjoy it, but you have to shift your diet around to keep it in balance. This woman was suddenly exercising far less often, yet eating just as much if not more, and adding the wine to help her relax because her normal relaxation technique (running) wasn't available to her. Now that she's been working with me, the weight is coming off. She still likes her glass of wine in the evenings, but when I explained that with 1:1:1 she would be down 30 pounds by the end of the year, even without running five days a week, she lit up. "I can do this!" she said.

Yet another client told me she'd been doing the Diabetes Diet.

"Do you have diabetes?" I said.

"No," she said. "I wish I did! Then maybe I'd stick to the diet."

Sometimes I just have to shake my head.

I've had clients tell me they wished they had celiac disease, dairy allergies, and thyroid issues; that they hoped they got the flu, diarrhea, or a stomach virus on their trip overseas. They wished all these maladies on themselves just to lose weight.

Why are we so desperate to get thin that we long for chronic diseases? When I worked at a bariatric clinic, I shared with a client the results of her metabolism test, and when I told her that she had a fast metabolism, she was crushed.

"I wanted a slow metabolism!" she moaned.

"Why?" I said.

"Because then I would have something to blame."

All of these clients were operating under false assumptions. They thought they could stick to an unsustainable way of eating and exercising, or they prioritized cheating over health, or they quit exercising and took in more calories and didn't understand why they gained weight. Or they got frustrated with slow and steady weight loss, not realizing that as the weeks pile up, so do the lost pounds. Even if you lose just 1 pound a week, you could be down 52 pounds by this time next year. That's a major accomplishment! They've all taught me a lot about how people think about food, and how what they intend to do

⓵⓵⓵

Start-Now Strategy

Think back to the times when you looked and felt your best. I don't mean the times when you lost weight but suffered because you didn't like the lifestyle. How were you eating, moving, and living when you felt strong, healthy, and slim? What were you feeling and thinking in those days? Who were you back then? What were you doing that you're not doing now? Can you reclaim some of those habits, to get that good feeling back? Thinking about the good old days can help get you back into the right state of mind for practicing a healthier lifestyle right now.

is often much different than what they actually do. That's been a valuable education for me.

My conclusion, after more than a decade as a nutritionist in private and clinical settings, is that people really are very confused. They honestly don't know how to eat anymore. They have lost their natural instincts. Hunger, satiety, the real taste of whole foods—these notions and instincts are disappearing. It's not that surprising, if you look at the way we live. The so-called information age might better be named the misinformation age. The media bombard us with constant messages that being fat is bad and worthy of ridicule and that being thin is good and makes people somehow superior. At the same time, restaurants serve huge portions of tempting food, so we've forgotten what a normal portion size is. We're full of guilt and cravings and hope and disappointment—no wonder people don't remember how to eat!

The good news is it's really not so hard to reclaim your natural instincts and get back into balance. You have those instincts inside of you right now. They're just buried under a bunch of ideas you should want to get rid of as much as you want to get rid of the extra pounds of fat you're carrying. You just have to get real. You have to face up to the fact that what you were doing before didn't work, and that most of the things you hear about weight loss simply aren't true—or aren't true for you.

It's time for a return to common sense, proportion, rationality, and eating like a normal person. *The One One One Diet* will show you exactly how to rebalance your diet so you can eat anything you want, just like those thin people you secretly envy. You might even learn to do it better, and with less anxiety, than those celebrities you admire. The formula is all you need to know.

But before we get into exactly how you can reclaim your natural tendencies to eat what your body actually needs to be thin, fit, and healthy, let's bust some very common diet myths.

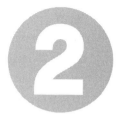

CHAPTER TWO

Myth Busting

N ow that I've got you thinking about whom to listen to when it comes to your health, I also want you to question the ideas you already have in your head. What's true and what's just a myth? My clients come in with all sorts of preconceived notions and I feel like half my practice is myth busting, so I would be remiss if I didn't bust some myths for you, too.

In that spirit, in this chapter I address the most prevalent dietary myths I've come across in my practice. I want you to understand why they aren't true and why you need to let go of these ideas right now, so you can finally reclaim the body you were meant to have. Are you ready to look truth squarely in the eye?

Myth #1: Gluten Is Bad

Let's just tackle this gluten issue right here, right now because this is one of those fads everyone's talking about these days. "Quit gluten! Quit wheat! Wheat gives you a big belly and chronic diseases and makes you obese and practically kills you the second you eat a slice of bread or a bite of pasta!"

Seriously, people.

You've heard that man cannot live on bread alone, but have you ever heard that man cannot live on bread? Not until this notion became a fad! You *can* live on bread, and even thrive, especially if it's made with good, natural, whole grains that supply all sorts of good nutrients your body needs, like protein, fiber, iron, and magnesium, and balanced with protein and fat.

My clients have a lot of questions about gluten, and so do the people I meet outside of my professional life. The other day, I was talking to a woman who works at my favorite French bakery. She told me she lost a lot of weight and was thrilled because she could now see her muscles. "How did you do it?" I asked.

"I cut out gluten and started doing yoga."

I couldn't help thinking about the breads and croissants and cookies and other beautiful French pastries in her bakery. If she cut out gluten, she couldn't enjoy any of them! Not even a thin slice of hot, crusty baguette! And for what? All because of a mistaken notion that giving up gluten will lead to weight loss (I'll explain why she likely lost weight in a minute). She could have chosen balance over restriction.

Going gluten-free is hot right now, probably because a few high-profile celebrities who can't or don't eat gluten have gone public and attributed their svelte figures to giving it up. But I feel sorry for gluten. It's a nutritious protein that comes from wheat, rye, and barley. It's the sticky, springy stuff that gives bread its chewy texture. Many meat alternatives like veggie burgers and veggie hot dogs are made with wheat gluten because when you remove the starch and knead it into its chewy form, it resembles the texture of meat. A lot of vegetarians eat it all the time because it's a great source of protein. It's true that some people can't eat it, just like some people can't eat strawberries or peanuts or drink milk, but for most healthy people, gluten is a perfectly safe and nutritious addition to the diet.

Okay, there is a kernel of truth to the wheat bashing: People eat way too much of it. You don't need 12 servings of wheat per day. That's completely out of balance. However, the idea that wheat is somehow evil, or genetically modified beyond recognition, or that it's so starchy you can't possibly stabilize your blood sugar if you eat it, and on and on and on is blatant exaggeration. Wheat has been a staple of the human diet for thousands of years and it contains protein and starch for energy. If you have a wheat allergy (which is rare) or celiac disease (which is also relatively rare), then yes, you should never, ever eat wheat or gluten. For most people, however, wheat fear is totally unfounded! Wheat is a perfectly fine and nutritious food, and cutting it completely out of your life will just make things more difficult.

Whether you're worried about wheat in general or gluten in particular, let me put your mind at ease. If you don't have a wheat allergy or celiac disease, you can eat wheat and gluten. On the 1:1:1 plan, wheat-based foods like bread, pasta, crackers, and anything made with flour, from bagels to birthday cake, count as a carb serving. You need carbs to fuel your brain and muscles, and wheat is a perfectly healthy one. In fact, many of the best sources of carbohydrate are made from wheat: whole grain bread, whole grain cereal, and whole grain crackers. Yes, a French bakery might not offer the most nutritious sources of gluten, but everyone who wants to enjoy an occasional croissant or baguette and doesn't have a medical problem should be able to.

Besides, giving up gluten is no path to weight loss, and could even lead to weight gain. A few studies even report nutritional deficiencies in

Food for **Thought**

According to the National Institutes of Health, about 1 of every 133 Americans has celiac disease. Celiac disease is a serious autoimmune disease that damages your small intestine. If you have it, you absolutely must not consume gluten. If you don't have it, however, gluten is probably just fine for you to eat. If it doesn't bother your stomach, take advantage of this protein in grain and enjoy it without guilt.

people on long-term gluten-free diets, especially among those who rely on a lot of packaged gluten-free foods. If you substitute gluten-free bread, cookies, tortillas, and cake for your gluten-containing favorites, you're going to be eating just as many carbs and just as much sugar. The only reason some people lose weight going gluten-free is because they eat more natural whole foods and they get their formerly excessive carbohydrate intake back into balance. That's all great, but you don't have to give up gluten to do it.

But what about the French baker who gave up gluten and lost weight? First of all, remember what I told you in the last chapter—this was *her experience,* not yours. Also, there are other likely explanations for why she lost weight. Here are some theories:

　　1. She has celiac disease. If this is true, gluten would be physically harmful to her (see box on page 21). I don't think it's likely, but it's possible.

　　2. She is now eating fewer carbs. Think about it—this woman works in a French bakery, so she was probably eating too many carbohydrates before she gave up gluten, and this could have put her out of balance.

　　3. It was really the yoga. Yoga could have increased her muscle mass so she burned more calories. Reducing stress can also help you to reduce compulsive stress eating.

All these factors worked for her, at least for now. But what if she decides to eat gluten again later? What if the temptations at work are too great? What if she genuinely misses the occasional French pastry? If she goes overboard on any starchy, sugary food (gluten-free or not), she will be out of balance and likely to gain back the weight.

Still unsure, because all those recent books targeting gluten and/or wheat sound so convincing? Think about it this way: Do you want to go through the rest of your life without pasta, birthday cake, cookies, toast, or a really good beer? Gluten-containing foods are comfort foods. They make us feel good inside. You should be able to eat food that makes you feel good.

Healthy eating is simply not an all-or-nothing kind of deal. Your choices aren't limited to (1) a totally gluten-free diet or (2) daily binges on pasta, bread, and cookies. You can live on the middle ground, and you should. Have your pasta, bread, cookie, or slice of birthday cake if you really want it, but let that one thing you want be your one carb in that meal or snack. The 1:1:1 plan will show you exactly how to do this.

Myth #2: Meat Is Bad, and Dairy Is *Really Bad*

Okay, let's knock out two myths in one. The other big food group that dieters tend to ban is animal products. Vegetarians don't eat meat, and vegans don't eat any animal products, including dairy products and honey. I have no problem with people who want to eat vegetarian or vegan for ethical reasons. For many people, animal welfare and environmental concerns are important, and they definitely are legitimate concerns. Many of the recent books singing the praises of a vegan or vegetarian diet make a lot of health claims. Although their advice is packaged as health or weight loss tips, their agenda is political. That's fine, but you should recognize it. A few studies have shown that vegetarians have lower blood pressure, lower cholesterol, and a lower risk of heart disease than meat eaters. I hear your arguments. But weight loss is not necessarily one of them.

That's not to say you can't eat this way and lose weight. Of course you can, and in fact 1:1:1 is perfectly compatible with these diets. Vegetarian and vegan diets include many nutritious choices that cover all the

Food for **Thought**

Need another reason to avoid the gluten-free aisle at your grocery store? How about the health of your bank account? According to the National Institutes of Health, gluten-free packaged foods are approximately 242 percent more expensive than their conventional, gluten-containing counterparts!

macronutrients you need (protein, carbs, fat). However, you can easily eat a junk-food diet and still technically be a vegan. I've met plenty of overweight and even obese vegetarians and vegans. It's not the stereotype because the reedy-looking celebrity vegans who write the books have careers that demand they stay in good shape. Cutting out meat and/or dairy is not the reason those people are thin. You can't just stop eating something and assume that's all you have to do.

Plenty of less-than-nutritious foods don't contain animal products. Think about vegetarian food choices. Many of them aren't lean at all. You could eat huge portion sizes of macaroni and cheese or nachos and still be vegetarian. Veggie chili loaded up with corn chips and avocados or a giant cupcake can be vegan. White bread, most types of sweeteners including high-fructose corn syrup, margarine, and fried potato and corn chips are all vegan. So are many brands of candy. You can also buy many highly

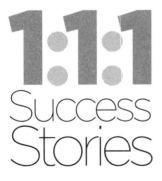

1:1:1 Success Stories

Name: **Heather Beeby**
Starting weight: **162 pounds**
Current weight: **134 pounds**
Height: **5'10"**

When I turned 30, I came to the harsh realization that my metabolism was not what it used to be. I decided that I needed to start working out and I gradually got up to 1½ to 2 hours of exercise a day, 6 days a week—boxing, kickboxing, P90X, and running. I always made time for a workout, no matter how busy I was at work or what fun things my friends had planned.

I did this for a year and I lost some weight, but I wasn't seeing the results I wanted. I kept reading in fitness magazines how optimum exercise results couldn't be achieved without the right diet. I thought I was eating in a healthy way, but I decided to consult a nutritionist. That was Rania. She asked me to keep a food log for a processed packaged vegan foods, from ice "cream" sandwiches to vegan bacon, and while some are slightly lower in fat or calories than the conventional versions, you might eat more of them because you think they're healthier. Many of these meat alternative products are also highly processed. Of course, on the 1:1:1 plan, you can eat anything you want, including veggie hot dogs and vegan cupcakes. There are no forbidden foods. But being vegan or vegetarian alone is not a weight loss strategy.

The bottom line is that you still need to stay in balance. You can't just cut out a food group and assume everything about your diet will be fine as long as you don't eat that one thing. That's not how it works. You can follow 1:1:1 just as well as any meat eater, and that's the key to balance, no matter what your dietary restrictions are.

And if you don't really want to eat that way but thought it would help you lose weight, rest easy. Animal products, especially organic grass-fed

---

week and then she reviewed it and made some tweaks. First she had me construct every meal according to 1:1:1. Then she pointed out where my portions were oversized. She never told me I couldn't eat something; she just gave me the tools to balance my choices. It was pretty easy.

What a difference! Within 4 months, I had lost 12 pounds and reached my goal weight of 150 pounds. I was ecstatic. I had no problem maintaining my weight loss for several months. But then I moved in with my boyfriend and my diet became unbalanced again. We went out for dinner and drinks a lot, and I liked it, but I gained 6 pounds in about 6 months. I wasn't willing to stop dining out, so Rania showed me how to apply 1:1:1 to my new lifestyle. Not only did it work, but it worked even better than the first time! In 10 weeks, I lost 22 pounds, and I've been at 134 ever since. I never feel deprived, and what I have learned is invaluable. I have never felt better about my health or my body, and 1:1:1 and Rania made this all possible.

meat and wild-caught fish, are rich in protein, bioavailable heme iron, and many other nutrients, including valuable omega-3 fatty acids. I totally get that you might not want to eat these foods, but don't give them up just to get skinny because you need lean protein, and animal products are an excellent source.

Now let's turn our attention to dairy. Sure, eating huge hunks of cheese or heaping bowls of ice cream isn't healthy and it's out of balance, not to mention very high in fat and calories, but you don't have to give up dairy altogether unless you have ethical or medical reasons to do so. You don't *need* dairy products to get protein and calcium, but they are an excellent source if you choose the right ones. For example, one of my favorite foods is low-fat Greek yogurt, which is very high in protein compared to conventional yogurt, with a rich, creamy texture. Cottage cheese can be a healthy snack or meal and a base for many delicious recipes. I often recommend string cheese as part of a healthy snack. You can even enjoy real cheese, real ice cream, and cream in your coffee, as long as you keep them in balance using 1:1:1. The same goes for eggs. Eggs are an excellent protein source, if you choose to eat them as part of your 1:1:1 strategy. They aren't required, but don't ban them just because you think they will make you fat.

If you object to the dairy and egg industries, fine. Just don't assume

Food for **Thought**

An easy way to balance a vegetarian or vegan diet is to eat a wide variety of vegetables and fruits, nuts, seeds, grains, and beans. Construct your meals according to 1:1:1, but switch them up often. Try vegetables you've never tried before. Try different grains, like millet, amaranth, quinoa, and buckwheat. Try different kinds of lentils and beans. Many ethnic cuisines have great vegetarian dishes. Try cooking meals from Mediterranean, South American, African, or Asian cultures for new, exciting flavors and healthful, nutritious meals.

you're going to be able to order that vegan T-shirt in extra-small because you cut meat, dairy, and eggs from your diet.

Myth #3: Pay Diet Plans Work Best

If I had a nickel for every client I've ever had who was a dropout from some pay diet plan, well, I'd have a lot of nickels. Paid diet plans are extremely popular, and part of the reason is that people believe if they pay for the diet, it will work. The theory goes that you won't want to waste your money, so you will do what the diet plan says, or that a diet plan that costs money must have more value and be more effective than a free diet plan (or no diet plan). But I've seen firsthand that in many cases, this is simply not true.

Whether you've enlisted with Weight Watchers or Jenny Craig or Nutrisystem or Medifast or eDiets or any of those in-person or online diet programs, you are likely to find that you are highly motivated—at first. When reality sets in and you get tired of eating the packaged foods or counting the points or not getting to have what you really want, that's when motivation flags. The camaraderie can be nice, but do you really need to pay for that?

Sure, some people really have lost a lot of weight on pay diet plans, and the diet plans are quick to plaster those people all over their advertisements (usually with a fine-print disclaimer underneath that says, "Results Not Typical"). Or they will pay some celebrity to do the diet plan and advertise the results. Maybe you even know someone who lost weight through a pay diet program. Those people are out there—but has anybody checked 2 or 3 years down the line? The percentage of people who keep the weight off is dismally small.

Every single diet out there has success stories, but my problem with these programs is that those fine-print disclaimers really are true: Losing weight and keeping it off through a pay diet program is *not a typical result*. Most people don't have that kind of success. They might lose weight, but most of the time, they gain it back. You really have to become a lifetime member if you want these programs to work, and a complicated system that tells you what to eat or has you counting points or eating packaged meals isn't sustainable over the long term, like a simple dietary strategy is. A study from UCLA that analyzed 31 long-term studies found that although people can often lose 5 to 10 percent of their body weight on any diet, most people regain the weight and then some within 4 to 5 years, and that dieting itself is actually a consistent predictor of future weight gain! How's that for a reason *not* to waste your hard-earned cash on tasteless frozen meals and counting points and going to meetings and obsessively posting on forums to talk about your successes and slipups? Do you want dieting to become your lifestyle?

I've met women in their fifties who have "done Weight Watchers" five times or more. Each time, they lose weight, and each time, they gain it back after they go off the program. Why keep doing that to yourself? If the plan was workable for life, you would never have to go off the plan at all. It would simply be the way you eat, and it would be easy, and you would enjoy it. (Which is exactly what the 1:1:1 plan is.)

I have a few other issues with these programs. For one thing, the people running them are usually not dietitians or nutritionists. They are just successful clients of the program. They have *experience,* but they don't have *expertise.* They might be able to inspire you in a peer-to-peer way, but how do you know they're telling you things that are actually healthy for you? Or that they are not on repeat mode, telling you the same thing they said to the woman in the previous meeting rather than something that will work for you personally?

Food for **Thought**

According to the Vegetarian Research Group, 7.3 million Americans are vegetarian, 1 million are vegan, and 22.8 million describe themselves as "inclined towards vegetarianism." The U.S. city with the most vegetarian restaurants is Portland, Oregon—the city where I live! Personally, I am not a vegetarian, but I don't eat meat at every meal.

Also, my clients have told me that when they were on a pay diet program, they did great, but they didn't know what to do when they went off it. They didn't learn anything. They followed the food plan exactly (or didn't and gave up), but once they didn't have that premade meal plan, they were lost. They didn't come away with any real, usable skills for eating in the real world.

Then you've got the humiliation factor—you go in and get weighed in front of everyone, and if you didn't lose weight, you feel so embarrassed. Who says healthy eating should be degrading? And don't even get me started about the quality of the packaged "food." Do you really want to give up eating real, fresh food? That's not healthy by any standard.

As for those celebrity endorsements—you know, the famous people who gained too much weight and then joined this or that program and got skinny again (at least for awhile)? Don't ever forget that they were paid to do that—reports say that Jessica Simpson got a $3 million contract to lose weight and endorse Weight Watchers. Studies show that when people are paid to lose weight, they're almost always more successful. I bet any of us could lose weight for a cool $3 million! But think about it: Getting paid is the exact opposite of what *you* do when *you* sign up for a pay diet plan. You pay *them*.

Wouldn't you rather be in control of your own weight loss and save your money for something more interesting, like a smaller size pair of skinny jeans? Or a whole new wardrobe?

Myth #4: Some People Will Never Be Able to Eat Normally

The crux of the 1:1:1 plan is that it helps you eat like a normal person again. This is exactly the opposite of what most diet plans do. They teach you that you *can't* eat normally if you want to lose weight. You have to restrict yourself, follow the plan, and go to meetings so you can all keep reminding each other that you can't eat like other people. There is this mentality that overweight and especially obese people have a special problem that requires a way of eating that's about as much fun as a medical prescription.

I say, nonsense!

Recently, my client, Patty, told me that her husband is thrilled that she finally eats like a normal person, now that she's working with me and eating according to 1:1:1. He's spent years watching her eat differently than the rest of the family, picking at salads or looking longingly at the french fries on his plate. Now she just eats what she wants because she has the tools to do it smartly. She loves that *he* loves that she can eat again—it's a big victory for someone who has struggled with food issues for years, and it's a big burden lifted off family members. Sometimes people don't realize that their diets and restrictions put stress on family members who don't understand them or feel they have to change the way they eat, too. The best part is that Patty is finally losing weight at a steady clip.

Myth #5: The U.S. Government Knows What You Should Eat

The U.S. government has been in the business of deciding what Americans should eat, beginning decades ago with the infamous Four Food Groups, then with the Food Pyramid, and now with its new ChooseMyPlate campaign (MyPlate.gov). The problem with the federal government dictating the food you put into your body is that it is advised by a bunch of people who make a lot of money selling you their particular kind of food—meat

Food for **Thought**

Weight Watchers overhauled its points system a few years ago, creating a new system called Points Plus. The purpose of the overhaul was to encourage healthier choices by making fruit free, but many members now report having more trouble losing weight. As a nutritionist, this makes sense to me. Fruit is a nutritious food to eat, but it is also high in natural sugars and is considered a carb choice on the 1:1:1 plan. If you eat a lot of it in addition to other carb choices, you will throw your diet out of balance. When you eat fruit at a meal or snack, it should be your only carb.

producers, dairy producers, and wheat producers. This doesn't necessarily mean the government has bad information, but it does mean profit is involved, and the result, in my opinion as a nutritionist, is that the recommendations are unbalanced and excessive.

According to the new MyPlate campaign, every meal should consist of fruit, vegetables, grains, protein, and dairy. That's a lot for one meal. You don't need that much food. You can benefit from eating all those food groups, but not at every meal. It's excessive. A meat, a grain, and a vegetable with butter or oil is a good meal. Imagine salmon with brown rice and steamed asparagus with butter. That's a great dinner. Why also add fruit and milk? Apple slices with peanut butter and a glass of milk make for a nice balanced snack. Why also add meat and vegetables? It's too much. Plus the MyPlate plan doesn't even mention fat, which is incredibly important for a healthy diet. Maybe the protein or dairy you choose will contain fat, or maybe you will put a fat such as olive oil on your vegetables, but the plan doesn't tell you to do so. Its message isn't clear, and it lends itself to abuse. Instead, follow 1:1:1 and you'll get balance in a sensible, moderate way, rather than stuffing yourself to fill the pockets of the food industries that have a serious financial stake in what the government tells you to eat.

Myth #6: Organic Food Is Diet Food

I had a client once who told me that she didn't understand why she wasn't losing weight because she was eating all organic. She'd read in a book that the chemicals in food make us fat, and that if you just eat organic, you won't be fat.

"What did you eat today for breakfast?" I asked.

She paused. "A quarter of an organic cherry pie."

Hmmm.

The word *organic* is seductive, but it's also misleading. *Organic* means a food is grown without pesticides or other chemicals and is not genetically modified. But it says absolutely nothing about the nutrient value of the food itself, or whether it's a good dietary choice, or whether it has excessive fat, sugar, or starch. A quarter of an organic pie for breakfast? That's not a healthy breakfast, even if it is a chemical-free breakfast. It

Start-Now Strategy

Instead of paying a diet plan, pay yourself! Start a bank account or get a piggy bank and pay yourself a certain number of dollars per pound you lose or goal you meet. Whether it is $1, $10, or $50 per pound, you could end up saving a lot of money for new clothes or even a vacation when you've reached your goal weight.

isn't balanced and it contains way too many calories, and too much sugar and fat for a single meal. (And very little protein.) Organic sugar is still sugar. Organic white flour is still white flour. Organic butter is still butter and organic lard is still lard. No wonder she wasn't losing any weight.

But chemicals scare people, so much so that they can forget what losing weight is really about. I had a woman come into my office recently who weighed 400 pounds. She sat down in the chair and looked me in the eye and said, "My biggest concern right now is plastic."

"Plastic?" I asked, not quite believing what I was hearing.

"Yes! Plastic. It leaches chemicals into food and poisons us."

This woman was at serious risk for catastrophic health problems, but she wasn't looking at what or how much she was eating. Instead, she was obsessing about what her food containers were made of. I do not in any way intend to belittle this woman's concern. She was an intelligent person, but she truly believed plastic was her biggest problem because she was misinformed.

I understand the concern. It's a toxic world. Many of my clients are concerned about the effects of toxins in foods and choose organic foods to avoid some of this chemical load. I think that's great, but it's not enough. Our environment is contaminated with chemicals and nobody can avoid them entirely. So while eating organic food may lighten your toxic load a bit, it's certainly no magic weight loss bullet—no, not even if the pie has whole wheat crust and the cookies were baked with agave nectar instead of sugar. Calories are calories, fat is fat, sugar is sugar, even when it comes without the pesticide sprinkles.

Myth #7: Food Can Heal You

The old Hippocrates adage to let food be thy medicine and medicine be thy food is quoted all the time in hundreds of diet books. However, this is only true to some extent. Food helps balance and sustain your body so it can heal most effectively on its own, but the food itself isn't fixing your medical problem, and a diet book should never replace a doctor. Food can help keep you healthy, and food can definitely make you sick, but it's not a cure-all.

A lot of books, websites, and people will tell you differently. They claim that this or that food is a "miracle cure," that this or that diet plan will treat or cure or at least "encourage healing" of all kinds of chronic diseases like cancer, diabetes, heart disease, celiac disease, allergies, even psychological problems. This is misleading, if not untrue.

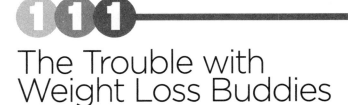

The Trouble with Weight Loss Buddies

If you join a group for people with "weight problems" you can get a lot of support, but there's a downside. It can make you all feel like there is something wrong with you, that you are different and can't eat normally. You don't have to be part of a diet group for this to happen—it often happens in groups of girlfriends who share a weight problem.

What if there's *nothing* wrong with you other than misinformation and a few bad habits? Get support when you need it, definitely, but go have fun with that group of friends trying to lose weight. Don't sit around comiserating about your food issues or worse, overeating together. Get out there and live your lives together instead.

We all know that eating more fish can improve your heart health, eating more fruits and vegetables can lower your cancer risk, and eating more fiber can help bring down high blood sugar levels. However, those foods aren't medicine. They're just healthy foods humans are meant to eat.

Have you noticed that most of these diets are pretty similar? They all emphasize healthful, nutrient-dense whole food. That's because this type of food will be more likely to give people all the nutrients they need. If you're allergic to a food (like milk or wheat) or have an autoimmune response to a food (as in celiac disease), then some foods can *hurt* you, but eliminating them doesn't *cure* you. It just takes away the damaging factor so natural healing can happen without interference.

Myth #8: Diet Food Helps You Lose Weight

Here's a crazy idea. If you're hungry, try eating *food*. And I mean real food. Not fake food.

Diet foods are fake foods—or more precisely, fake "foods." Manufacturers use all kinds of food-processing tricks and chemicals to trick you into thinking you just ate a blueberry pie or a chocolate eclair or a regular cola, when all you really ate was artificial sweetener, filler, even wood pulp. Remember when I said that on the 1:1:1 plan, no food is forbidden? I meant no *food* is forbidden. The fake stuff should be totally off your menu and out of your kitchen.

If you eat this stuff, your brain might be fooled for a few minutes, but your body won't be fooled for long. Fake foods cause all kinds of trouble in your body. Artificial sweetener, whether in yogurt or diet soda or something else, can actually disrupt your body's natural insulin cycle. Researchers at the Washington University School of Medicine in St. Louis tested 17 severely obese people to see how their blood sugar and insulin would respond to artificial sweeteners. When study subjects drank sucralose (a common artificial sweetener) before a glucose challenge test, they had higher blood sugar peaks and a 20 percent higher insulin level than when they drank water before the test. As you may know, high blood sugar and excessive insulin production are conditions that may lead to diabetes. That diet soda you drink with your meal might be doing you more harm than good!

Fillers and chemicals that mimic natural flavors have similar effects. Your body feels full temporarily, but because it isn't getting the nutrients that should coincide with a full feeling, it gets confused and you end up hungrier. Also, many processed foods contain trans fats (vegetable fats chemically treated to become similar to saturated fats, which increases shelf life in processed food). Many studies have clearly demonstrated that trans fats damage your heart and arteries much more than saturated fat. (You can tell when a food contains trans fat if you see the words "partially hydrogenated' in the ingredients list.) Other fake fats meant to pass right through the digestive system without being absorbed (and therefore without adding any calories or fat to your body) are infamous for causing intense gastrointestinal distress in many people. You may also end up eating way too much since you think the fat doesn't count.

Then there are all those "fat-free" foods. Studies show that where a person might eat one real cookie, he or she is more likely to eat 10 fat-free cookies. That results in a calorie overload, not a calorie deficit.

As a nutritionist, I hate to see this kind of overeating, especially of fake food. Instead, just eat the real food, using the 1:1:1 strategy. It'll taste better, be more satisfying, and make you feel like you're eating normally.

Start-Now Strategy

Here's a good way to go organic on the cheap: head out to your local farmers' market! Many small, local farms don't use chemicals even though they might not be able to afford an organic certification. Ask the farmer about his pesticide use—a luxury you don't get when you shop at a supermarket! Farmers are usually happy to tell you all about their methods, as well as give you ideas for how to use the produce they sell. See what's in your area and stock up on yummy vegetables through the whole growing season—and hold the chemicals.

Myth #9: You Have to Start on a Monday

Monday holds such promise. It's a new beginning. A do-over for all the dietary mistakes you made last week. However, Monday's promise is a false promise. It implies you are starting something you will eventually stop, so why start at all? Monday is just another day—and another excuse.

People like to mark a day to begin something, but what are you beginning? Giving up your favorite foods or starting a restrictive diet? That's nothing to celebrate. Most diets don't involve sustainable behaviors. They involve drastic, temporary measures to help you lose weight, but starting them on Monday (or any other day) just means that on some future date— probably Thursday or Friday—you're going to go back to your old ways.

You don't ever have to start a diet, let alone go off one, and you certainly don't need to wait until Monday to start eating right. Instead, starting right now, eat what you love, make good choices most of the time, and remember 1:1:1. Once you change your permanent eating habits, Monday will be just another day. It won't lie to you, and it won't abandon you on Friday. And you won't need it. Because you will have moved on.

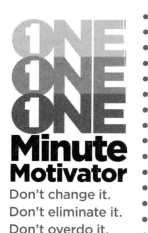

One One One Minute Motivator

Don't change it.
Don't eliminate it.
Don't overdo it.
Just moderate it.

Myth #10: But You Can Just Have Surgery!

Stop! Freeze! Back away from the surgical theater! A lot of people seek bariatric surgery, especially since many insurance companies now cover the procedure. That sounds like "free" dramatic weight loss, right? It sounds like the easy way.

I can assure you, it's *not* the easy way. Going under the knife is an extreme solution to a problem much more easily tackled with lifestyle changes. It includes major risks, including death, and some people end up gaining the weight back anyway. There are no guarantees with bariatric surgery. It's a procedure best left to those in serious, imminent danger from morbid obesity. In my opinion, there's a reason why the initials of bariatric surgery are "BS."

I spent years working as a nutrition consultant for a bariatric surgery clinic that's helped many people who really needed it, so I'm not knocking bariatric surgery across the board. However, some of the people I met who intended to have bariatric surgery ended up opting out because the 1:1:1 strategy was so effective that they lost weight without the surgery—and without the risks. This is what I loved to see. A lot of my clients also told me they'd lost 100 pounds or more before, but gained it back, so now they wanted to get rid of those pounds with surgery. I told them, "If you've lost 100 pounds before, you can do it again. You don't need this radical approach. Do it this time so it sticks. Do it with 1:1:1."

Also remember that when you lose weight on your own without surgical intervention, you won't have scars, you won't have any permanently altered internal organs, and you won't risk death. It's time for a reunion with common sense, not a first date with a scalpel.

But, But, But . . .

Everyone is full of opinions, and everyone is full of excuses. I know. I think I've heard them all. After working with hundreds of clients over the years, I know how human beings tick. I understand. But you aren't going to get anywhere with your weight loss effort if you keep fooling yourself. It's time to take a good, hard look at what people are really telling you, so you can understand why weight loss hasn't worked in the past, or why it worked for awhile, then stopped working. You need to understand why you gained all the weight back.

Here's my radical notion: Stop. Just stop. Stop the diets. Stop the food plans. Stop the crazy food rules and restrictions. Stop forbidding entire food groups. Stop the public weigh-ins. Stop telling yourself that food is bad. Stop depriving yourself of pleasure.

Food is good. It nourishes you and makes you feel alive. That's how it should be. That's the simple truth. You just need to know how to eat it.

CHAPTER THREE

Balancing Act

Want to know how to get out of a false diet mentality? Understand what food is and what it can do for you so you make smart decisions about what to eat. Yes, pleasure should be part of it. You should definitely enjoy your food and choose foods you love, but the more you know about nutrition, the better you'll be able to choose from the huge variety of available foods out there.

This chapter will introduce you to the concept of balance, because balancing your intake of the three essential macronutrients—protein, carbohydrates, and fat—is the key to making food work for you and the key to 1:1:1.

Protein, carbohydrates, fat. They're a perfect trio with thousands of different possible combinations. Each one of those nutrients is found in hundreds of foods, and each is important for your health. None of them is bad. Seriously! Fat is not bad. Carbs are not bad. Protein is not bad. There is no bad real food, despite what you might've heard or read. This is the ultimate and final myth I want to bust: *No food is good or bad.*

The only thing "bad" in a diet is excess or deficiency. The only thing "good" in a diet is balance. Period.

So let's get specific. If you think fruit is good—or bad—or that meat is bad—or good—or that white flour is bad and whole wheat flour is good, or that sweet potatoes are good but white potatoes are bad, or that all fat or all protein or all carbohydrates are either *bad bad bad* or *good good good,* then you've probably been told some lies. They're all just foods, with different combinations of nutrients. Some are better for some purposes than others, but in general, these foods are all fuel for your body, and they all contain different combinations of nutrients your body needs.

Okay, I know what you're thinking. An apple is better than a candy bar, a bag of baby carrots is better than a bag of potato chips, and a glass of water is better than a soda. I see your point, so let me rephrase. An apple is more nutritious and fiber rich than a candy bar. On the other hand, depending on the brand—a Snickers, perhaps?—the candy bar may have more protein. There is nothing wrong with having a candy bar once in a while. If you need protein, you might prefer the candy bar over the apple. Just have the mini size, to keep your portion under control.

As for the baby carrots versus the potato chips, sure. Baby carrots have more fiber, less fat, and more vitamins, but that doesn't mean you can't sometimes choose the potato chips. Just have 1 ounce and choose the baby carrots more often. The potato chips aren't "bad." They're just not the *best* choice from a nutritional standpoint. But from an emotional standpoint? Sometimes only the chips or the candy will do. Just count those as your one carb for that one meal or snack, and be content knowing you're still in balance.

The problem is, too many diet plans out there tell you that one of the three essential macronutrients (the primary nutrients your body needs to function: protein, carbohydrates, and fats) is more important or more dangerous than the other two. "Eat more protein but no carbs! Eat more carbs but no fat! Eat more fat but no protein!" All of these methods are out of balance, unless they're helping to correct an already out-of-balance diet. For example, if you eat too many carbs and not enough protein, you can benefit from eating more protein, but you don't want to cut carbs completely out of your life. No way! Just balance them with the protein and fat, and you'll be fine. Any other method might result in temporary weight loss (mostly of water weight), but not long-term weight loss, and it probably won't be sustainable over the long term.

Furthermore, not only do these notions knock you out of balance, but they can actually cause physical harm. You need protein, but overdoing it can make you sick, stress your kidneys, and put excessive strain on your digestive system. You need carbohydrates, but too many can pile on the calories, causing weight gain, and simple carbs like white flour and sugar can lead to inflammation, which in turn can lead to chronic diseases. You need fat, but too much can clog your arteries and cause excess weight gain. Not enough, on the other hand, can lead to dry skin, hair, and nails; poor mood; and a metabolism that holds on to every bit of fat you eat as a survival mechanism.

Your body isn't a mad scientist's lab. You shouldn't be messing around like that, experimenting on yourself to see how long you can go without an essential nutrient. You really honestly could make yourself sick, or worse. Just eat in balance. It's safe, it's tested, it's proven, and it's the most natural way for humans to eat.

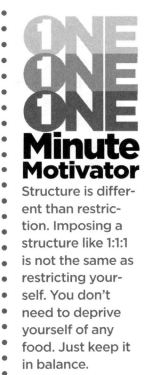

ONE 1 ONE 1 ONE Minute Motivator

Structure is different than restriction. Imposing a structure like 1:1:1 is not the same as restricting yourself. You don't need to deprive yourself of any food. Just keep it in balance.

The Logic behind 1:1:1

People often ask me if 1:1:1 is based in science, and the answer is a resounding yes! You don't need any fancy studies, however, to show you why 1:1:1 works. Nutritional science has known for many years that humans need a balance of protein, carbohydrates, and fat to stay healthy, but many fad diets restrict one of these macronutrients in a way that can lead to hunger, depressed metabolism, crazy blood sugar levels, and feelings of deprivation. The 1:1:1 plan is a return to sanity based on nutritional science. However, I would like *you* to fully understand why it works where many other diet plans don't.

• **The 1:1:1 plan naturally limits calories.** We all know the old saying: Weight loss is just a matter of eating less and exercising more. While this is an oversimplification, the fact is if you eat fewer calories without changing anything else, you'll lose weight. It's simple math. If you burn 3,500 more calories than you eat over the course of a week, you'll lose a pound.

A recent randomized controlled study from Switzerland compared people eating calorie-restricted diets for 12 weeks. The difference was that one group ate a low-GI diet and the other a high-GI diet. Both groups lost equal amounts of weight, suggesting that the calorie restriction, not the GI of the foods, led to weight loss. You might think, "Well, I'll just cut back on calories. Who needs 1:1:1?" You do! The problem with most calorie-restricted diets is that they leave people feeling deprived, and that leads to what doctors call "compliance issues." *Compliance* means the patient sticks to the prescription. If you don't stick to your diet—if you are noncompliant—then it's not going to work.

The 1:1:1 plan is an elegantly simple way to restrict calories while eliminating feelings of deprivation, so you can stick to it forever! Because you can choose any food you want, within the 1:1:1 framework, it's not a diet you go on and go off. It's a lifestyle that naturally keeps your calorie count under control.

• **The 1:1:1 plan naturally balances your blood sugar.** The food you eat gets transformed into glucose in your bloodstream. This triggers your body to release insulin, which sweeps up the blood sugar and shuttles it into the muscles and organs where it can be used for energy. This system works—unless you eat too much, or eat in an imbalanced way. In particular, eat too many simple carbs (like bread and pasta) and/or too much sugar (like candy and cupcakes), and your blood sugar level will rise too high, causing your body to release excessive insulin, which can lower your blood sugar too much, making you feeling ravenous again—after you just ate too much! Riding this blood sugar roller coaster too often can also desensitize your body to the effects of insulin. Eventually, this can result in metabolic syndrome, a prediabetic condition.

Avoiding big swings in blood sugar is obviously important for avoiding diabetes in your future, but in the short term, it's also important for appetite control. When your blood sugar is steadier, you don't get so hungry, which means you have an easier time controlling your eating. The 1:1:1 plan naturally keeps blood sugar steady because you always combine protein and fat with carbs, which slows the release of blood sugar into your system so your body can use less insulin.

• **The 1:1:1 plan naturally keeps your metabolism running strong.** Because you eat five times a day on 1:1:1, your body stays busy digesting food during the day, when you're most active. That keeps your metabolism humming. Limiting excessive carbohydrate intake and eating fat with every meal also keeps your body in fat-burning mode.

• **The 1:1:1 plan provides a diversity of macronutrients and micronutrients.** If you tend to eat mostly carbs or protein or fat, you're likely to be deficient in one or more macronutrients, as well as the many micronutrients you'd get from a more diverse diet. Because 1:1:1 forces you to stay creative by choosing a protein, carb, and fat with every meal, you're more likely to get a wider range of micronutrients, which is healthier for you and keeps your body working more efficiently.

• **Eating frequently on the 1:1:1 plan keeps you satisfied.** People often get hungry on calorie-controlled diets. But because you eat five times a day on 1:1:1, you won't get hungry. It's always almost time for another meal or snack! The satiety and satisfaction you get from these frequent meals will keep you from wanting to eat more than your body needs and keep you from obsessing about food all day.

• **The 1:1:1 plan puts you in control.** If you go on a diet and the diet tells you what to eat, the diet is in control of you. People don't tend to like that. This is where the psychological benefit of 1:1:1 comes into play. Nobody is telling you what to do. *You* are the one empowered to decide what you want to eat. The 1:1:1 plan puts you back in charge of your diet, so you're no longer at the mercy of food or somebody else's meal plan. It's all about you—just as it should be, because it's your body and your life.

All this general knowledge is well and good, but it can also be beneficial to understand some specifics, like what happens when you eat too much healthy food, or too little, or too much or too little of any one macronutrient. Let's look at those issues now.

Too Much Good Stuff

You know you need nutrients, and what many of my clients tend to do is get them all—and then some! When you overeat any food, including those that are nutritious and generally considered healthful food choices, you can still foil your weight loss. Our food-obsessed culture has ways of fattening up just about everything, even vegetables, with heavy dips and deep-fat frying, or by drizzling butter all over them. Not that we eat very many vegetables—but even when we do, we tend to fry them or drown them in oil. (French fries are one of the three most commonly consumed vegetables among 9- to 11-month-olds . . . yikes!) Very few people binge on kale or green beans, but batter-dipped deep-fried green beans or onion rings? Absolutely.

Even more often, I see people overeating "health foods," such as whole grain bread and pasta, sweet fruit, fatty nuts and avocados, sweet potatoes, and organic meat. These are all healthful foods and sound virtuous, but too much of any of them can still contribute to a weight problem.

Just imagine this super politically correct, health-nut dinner: a heaping bowl of quinoa pasta with organic free-range, gluten-free turkey meatballs and artisanal Parmesan cheese imported from Italy; a crusty whole grain baguette from a local bakery with extra virgin olive oil; a huge salad of fresh local greens, cherry tomatoes, raw goat cheese from a local dairy, and avocados from the farmers' market drizzled with homemade vinaigrette; and a glass of sulfite-free organic wine, with a square of fair-trade extra-dark chocolate for dessert.

Guess what? It's too much good stuff. You could have any of those things (like a serving of pasta with meatballs and cheese, or a salad with goat cheese and avocados and a glass of wine), but having them *all* is overdoing it by a long shot. This meal has multiple protein, carb, and fat servings, and if you eat like this all the time, you're probably going to gain more weight than you'd like. Likewise, imagine eating slice after slice of fresh, hot whole grain bread straight out of the oven with real dairy butter. Imagine eating a box of fiber-rich vegan cookies. Or a big fruit salad made with a whole banana, a bunch of grapes, slices from a whole orange, a whole cubed apple, and a whole mango. Or a bowl of steaming hot oatmeal with almonds and blueberries and raisins and cinnamon and raw honey and organic cream.

Every one of these meal or snack ideas is out of balance.

This is why you can eat in a way you think is totally healthy and still be overweight. On the flip side, this is also why you can be at your ideal weight, healthy and fit, and still eat "bad" foods. A few strips of bacon every once in a while, the occasional dessert on a holiday, a glass of wine or a cocktail after dinner, a sandwich with white bread, a small order of french fries every now and again—all are fine choices if you keep them in proportion.

This is what it means to eat normally. You don't eat too much "good stuff" (meaning the foods everybody thinks are healthful), but you don't eat too much "bad stuff" either (meaning all those foods people feel guilty about). You can eat anything you want and reach and stay at a healthy weight when you keep your intake in balance with the other food choices you make.

Not Enough Good Stuff

Just as some people tend to eat too much "good stuff," some also tend not to eat enough "good stuff." They may only eat the few foods they like without thinking about nutrition at all, or they decide to severely limit one of the three categories. People need a certain amount of food to have enough energy to function. That means that in limiting one nutrient category, you are by necessity likely to overeat the other categories. And that's why mistaken notions about the relative "badness" of a food category can really mess with your health.

For example, let's say you have the idea that carbs are bad. Maybe you've been on low-carb diets before and they worked, and you can't get it out of your head that the shiny red apple in the fruit bowl—not to mention something as sinful as bread or pasta—is going to make you fat! You wouldn't be the first to operate and eat under that false assumption. However, if you strictly limit your carbohydrate intake, you not only won't get enough carbohydrates—which can translate to not enough energy for your brain and muscles—but you'll probably get too much protein and fat. This can result in high cholesterol, clogged arteries, high blood pressure, stressed kidneys, low energy, sallow skin, and bad breath. Not exactly attractive.

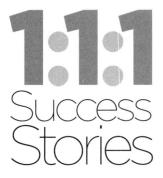

1:1:1 Success Stories

Name: **Stacy England**
Starting weight: **260**
Current weight: **200**
Height: **5'10"**

When I look back at photos of myself in high school and early college, I can see now that I was at an average body weight, but back then I always felt that I was too heavy. I don't think it helped that I am very tall, so when other girls were talking about wanting to weigh 115 and I weighed 150, I felt huge—but in reality I looked great. That's a healthy weight for me.

I think I really started gaining in college—you know, those freshman 15—and it just spiraled from there. The highest weight I saw on the scale was just over 260. I probably weighed more at some points. Sometimes I just refused to weigh myself. I stayed between 250 and 260 for a few years. I kept going to school (getting a master's and currently working on my doctorate) while also working several jobs. I sometimes overate out of exhaustion and definitely made poor food choices when I was too tired to cook. I would also find myself reaching for sweets as a way to relax or as a reaction to being overstressed. I believe many of my problems with overeating were connected to emotions.

If you think protein is bad, you'll have just as many problems. Maybe you've read a few books on veganism and you now avoid animal products like the plague. Many vegetarians and vegans also avoid soy because they know that overeating processed soy foods comes with its own list of potential health problems (like thyroid issues or hormone imbalance). However, if you shun meat and fish, eggs and milk, even soy, then you could become deficient in protein, which provides your body with the substance to build muscle, repair organs, produce healthy skin, hair, and nails—even maintain healthy bones. Plus you're probably going to get too many carbohydrates and too much fat. A lot of my vegetarian and

---

At my heaviest, I could just feel that this wasn't me. I like to be spontaneous, have fun, try new things. My weight was limiting. I exceeded the safe weights to kayak or skydive. I couldn't go shopping with the girls because I'd have to go to specialty stores. I love to travel but worried each time about whether or not I would be asked to buy an extra seat on the plane. I began to feel like my weight was a barrier to living the kind of life I wanted to live.

Now that I eat according to 1:1:1, I feel great. I have more energy, I feel more confident and in control, my skin is clearer, and I don't feel deprived in any way. In one year, I have lost 60 pounds! I think more about the protein, carb, and fat ratio of everything I eat, and I'm much more mindful about my choices. My meals used to be very carb-heavy and now I understand how to keep carbs in balance. The food log feedback was very helpful to me, and so was the way Rania coached me on stress reduction techniques. I don't like to cook so Rania gave me ideas for foods that were extremely easy to prepare, and once I realized that I didn't have to do major cooking to be healthy, I found that I actually didn't mind cooking about once a week—not because I have to but because now I am motivated to eat less processed food. I want to feel good and be in control of my life, and that's exactly what's happened with 1:1:1.

vegan clients have this problem. They overeat carbohydrates and gain a lot of weight quickly, and they say they're always hungry. It's a frustrating way to feel when you think you are doing the right thing.

If you think fat is bad, you could become deficient in it. When this happens, your hair and skin will dry out and your nails will crack. You will look older. (Eek!) You could even experience memory problems and depression. Plus, you will be more likely to overeat carbohydrates and protein. I have clients who have been on low-fat or no-fat diets who gorge on fat-free cookies and fat-free coffee creamer and other fake foods as well as huge bowls of pasta or bread without butter, and they can't understand why they don't feel well (and can't lose weight). Fat makes you feel fuller and more satisfied, helps keep your blood sugar level stable when you eat carbs, and also helps you absorb a lot of the vitamins from fruits and vegetables that could otherwise pass right through your system, unused.

You need all three, period. Now let's look briefly at why each one is so important. I'm going to put on my nutritionist cap now, but I'll try not to get too science-y on you.

Protein Is Power

Protein is absolutely essential to growth, rebuilding, healing, and strength. Protein is what the body uses to build muscle and repair tissues that have broken down, either from heavy exercise (like weight lifting), injury, or just living and aging.

When you eat protein, your body breaks it down into the amino acids it needs to maintain itself. Some of these amino acids are essential, meaning your body can't make them so you need to obtain them from food. You can get enough of these essential amino acids by eating a serving of protein with every meal or snack. Without that, your body will start breaking down muscle to get the protein it needs, which will make you weaker, slow your metabolism, and make you gain fat and weight faster. It's very important to keep a steady supply of protein coming in. Protein also keeps you from getting overly hungry—it's a natural appetite suppressant. Great for you overeaters, right? Protein helps dampen excessive eating in another way, too. When you eat it with carbs, it slows down the rate at which your body digests the carbs and feeds glucose into the bloodstream. This helps to keep your blood sugar in a steady state, without the surges and drops that can make you feel crazy and binge-eat. (I'll explain more about this in the carbohydrate section, so stay tuned!) This is why you should never eat carbohydrates alone. You should *always* enjoy them with protein and fat.

However, you don't need as much protein as some diet books or programs might lead you to believe. The human body can digest only about 30 grams of protein in one meal—that's about a 4-ounce hamburger patty or steak, or a 3½-ounce chicken breast. People on low-carb diets or paleo diets are likely to eat more than this, taxing the digestive system as it tries to pass half of that big steak through without using the protein.

In fact, too much protein can cause a lot of problems. One of my clients, a former athlete named Dave, was always a big, muscular guy, but he shot up to 275 pounds after graduating from college, when he began working long hours and stopped exercising. A low-carb diet sounded appealing to him because he loved steak, bacon, cheese, and a big plate of eggs and sausage, so he went from eating doughnuts for breakfast and sandwiches for lunch to eating eggs and bacon for breakfast and burgers without the bun for lunch—hold the fries. He quickly lost 30 pounds.

The problem was that Dave's total cholesterol level shot up to 245 mg/dl and his doctor warned him that he could be headed for a heart attack. He began to doubt the efficacy of his low-carb lifestyle. Then he started

Food for **Thought**

A study published in the *British Medical Journal* reported that among 43,396 Swedish women aged 30 to 49, low-carb, high-protein diets were associated with increased risk of cardiovascular disease.

to miss beer. One day, he had a beer, and then he couldn't stop eating carbs. He began bingeing on nachos, pizza, and giant plates of spaghetti. His body was desperate for carbohydrates because it was out of balance. When he came to see me, he had gained back all the weight he lost plus 25 more pounds. He was up to 300 pounds! It was hard for him to accept at first that he didn't have to go back to the low-carb lifestyle, until I reminded him what it had done to his cholesterol level. He decided to give 1:1:1 a try, and now he's down 80 pounds! At 220 pounds, he's motivated and on his way to his goal weight of 195.

Low-carb diets have other ill effects. For one thing, the hunger-dampening effects of protein can go too far, so that you skip vitamin-rich foods like fruits and vegetables. Also, protein doesn't have fiber—that's why you need grains, fruits, and vegetables along with it. Otherwise, you might get constipated (no thanks!). Too much protein in the absence of carbohydrates can also give you bad breath and make you irritable (carbs tend to have that feel-good effect).

Finally, diets that promote too much protein at the expense of other foods are extremely hard to maintain. Life without sandwiches, pizza, pasta, or dessert? You might ask yourself, "Do I really have to eat another boring chicken breast tonight?" It can take all the fun out of meals, which you're likely to enjoy much more if you have more variety—a protein, a carb, and a fat.

The deprivation factor is why so many people (like Dave) lose weight at first on low-carb diets, but then give up, binge on carbohydrates, and end up gaining back more weight than they lost. It can also make you do some wacky things. Another low-carb client, Dara, was on a plan that allowed just 20 grams of carbs a day, and she proudly told me she'd figured out how many carbs were in her favorite candy: M&Ms. She would eat 33 M&Ms every day, plus meat. That was it. No grains, no vegetables, no fruit. She couldn't understand why she was having what I referred to as "the M&Ms"—moodiness and muscle aches! When I explained that she could still have M&Ms but she needed to include other carbs and add some vegetables to her diet, she agreed to try it. (As long as I didn't forbid those M&Ms!) Dara is now down 15 pounds. Many of my ex-low-carbers, who forgot how to eat normally, bounced back to a balanced mode when they switched to the 1:1:1 plan and kick-started their weight loss again.

1:1:1 doesn't prioritize protein, but it doesn't marginalize protein either. It puts protein exactly where it should be: in balance. It's much simpler, more rational, easier, and you'll never feel deprived of anything you wish you could have—not bacon, not burgers, not even Buffalo wings.

Carbohydrate Conundrum

Carbs are what dieters—especially women—tend to overeat the most. For whatever biochemical, psychological, or habitual reason, a lot of my female clients find themselves in a love affair with carbs: bread, pasta, potatoes, or sugar in all its wonderful forms (candy, ice cream, cookies, pancakes, frozen yogurt, giant muffins paired with syrupy lattes topped with whipped cream).

Just as our bodies need protein, our bodies definitely need carbohydrates. They're the body's primary source of energy. Here's how it works: When your body digests carbohydrates, they get converted into glucose, which is routed into your bloodstream. Your muscles and organs need glucose to function—it provides quick energy and the fuel that runs your body. To help get the glucose where it needs to be, your body releases insulin, which shuttles the glucose into the right places. Excess gets stored in the liver and muscles as glycogen, for when you'll need it—like

Food for **Thought**

Twenty different amino acids build protein. If a food has all 20, it's called a complete protein. If it doesn't have all 20, it is an incomplete protein. Examples of complete proteins include meat, poultry, fish, milk, eggs, and soy products. Examples of incomplete proteins are most nuts, grains, legumes, and vegetables. Quinoa is one of the few grains that is a complete protein.

a spare gas tank. It's a great system, unless you flood your body with so much glucose that it doesn't have places to send it all. Your liver can only store so much, and your muscles and organs only need so much at a time. So guess where the excess blood sugar goes. It gets converted to fat. Fat, fat, fat. People tend to think that fat makes you fat, but for most people these days, it's excessive carbohydrates.

If you keep going, keep pumping carbs into your system beyond your body's needs, the situation can get even worse. When you get too much glucose, your body can't take it all in so it keeps running freely through the blood—this can be dangerous, causing excessive thirst, urination, fatigue, dry mouth, blurred vision, flushing, increased heart rate, weak pulse, and vomiting. Your body will pump out extra insulin to try to handle the extra blood sugar but eventually can lose its sensitivity to insulin, and this is what can lead to diabetes. When insulin stops working well, blood sugar will get even more out of control, and the chronic overeating of carbs will just keep making the situation worse. You'll get fatter and sicker.

But don't let this scare you away from carbs! In balance, carbs are extremely important for energy. As long as you balance your carbohydrates with protein and fat to slow down that blood sugar surge, you can have your carbs and eat them, too. Choose nutrient-rich carbs like fruit and whole grains most of the time, but feel free to indulge in the occasional refined carbohydrate choice. Just remember, you only get one. Pick the carb you want the most—the bread or the pasta or the dessert or glass of wine. Never all four.

A lot of my clients have trouble losing weight because of carbohydrates. I remember one client, a lawyer in her thirties named Sandra, who was very detail oriented and obsessively diligent about her work. She couldn't understand why the one thing in her life she couldn't seem to control was her weight. When I looked at her food journal, the problem was obvious. She was eating low-carb all day. She would typically have an egg white omelet with vegetables for breakfast and a salad with chicken, hold the croutons, for lunch. She would snack on carrots and celery, then go to the gym and do an hour-long spin class after work. By the time dinner rolled around, she thought she could splurge because she'd been so "good" and she would have pasta, bread, wine, and dessert. She figured she would burn it all off and deserved to splurge, but she was actually undoing all her efforts throughout the day. She wasn't eating carbs when she needed them the most (before her workout, for energy), and she was eating too many of them when she needed them the least (right before bedtime).

Actually, nighttime is the worst time to eat carbs because that's just the time of day when you *don't* need a lot of quick energy. You need carbs during the day. Your brain and your muscles require carbohydrates, so when you don't eat them all day, you get tired, you get cravings, and you don't have as much energy as you need. (I'll talk more about the supercharged technique of going lower-carb at dinner only in Chapter 7.)

Of course, carb issues go in both directions. I have a vegan client, Lucy, who thought she was eating really well all the time. She couldn't understand why she was overweight. She read the book *Skinny Bitch* and told me that the book said she would be skinny if she became a vegan.

Food for **Thought**

The glycemic index (GI) is a measure of how quickly blood glucose levels rise after eating a particular food. Knowing this number can be helpful if you're eating a carb by itself. High-GI carbs include white bread, white rice, most cereals, white potatoes, soda, and candy. Low-GI carbs include whole wheat pasta, bran cereal, lentils, and whole fruits (especially orchard fruits and berries). However, the good news for people following the 1:1:1 plan is that even high-GI carbs will become lower GI when combined with protein and fat, because both protein and fat help slow the release of glucose into the bloodstream. Score another one for 1:1:1!

So why did she weigh 200 pounds and look nothing like those cartoon girls on the cover?

When I looked at her food diary, I saw that for breakfast, she was eating a big bowl of oatmeal or cereal with fruit, dry toast with organic jam, and orange juice. For lunch she was having rice and beans with corn or pasta salad, and for dinner, she was having more pasta or rice with vegetables, fruit for dessert, maybe wine, and maybe a vegan cupcake. Her snacks were whole grain pretzels, rice cakes, low-fat vegan cookies, or fruit, such as a banana or grapes.

Lucy's meals were almost solely made of carbohydrates. She was getting very little protein or fat, and she was hungry all the time so she snacked constantly. She's not only an example of someone eating "too much good stuff," but of someone eating way too many carbs. Most of the individual choices she was making were fine on their own, but put together, they'd thrown her way out of balance.

Fabulous Fat

Dieters tend to be fat-phobic. The idea that fat makes you fat peaked in the 1980s and resulted in a low-fat craze, and I thought we'd be over all of that by now, but a lot of people still fear fat. A few popular diet plans still shun fat, and some people claim a low-fat diet is best for heart health. Of course, I'm not going to tell you to disobey your doctor! If your doctor advises that you follow a low-fat diet, that's what you should do. However, for most people, fat is not just yummy. (Butter! Olive oil! Heavy cream! Peanut butter!) It's absolutely essential.

Although it sounds counterintuitive, your body can't effectively burn fat if you aren't eating enough fat. Eating fat also triggers the release of a hormone called leptin that signals your brain that you've had enough food, which helps you stop eating sooner and stay full longer. (Leptin production may not work as well in obese people, and lack of sleep is also known to inhibit leptin production.) The essential fatty acids in certain dietary fats (for example, in salmon, walnuts, and olive oil) help your body to absorb vitamins and metabolize your food, and actually improve heart health. Fat, like protein, also helps to slow the release of glucose into the bloodstream from carbohydrates and helps moderate insulin secretion so your blood sugar and insulin levels stay more stable. Fat is a source of energy, and it makes your skin supple and your hair shiny. Fat is also very important for memory and mood. It makes you feel content. You need fat.

But too much fat isn't good for you, either. It can clog your arteries, eventually making them less flexible, which can lead to high blood pressure. Fat is also higher in calories per gram than either protein or carbs, so too much fat can lead to weight gain. One almond has 8 calories, and that doesn't seem like very much, but what if you eat a couple of handfuls a day? You could easily eat 800 or even 1,000 calories just in almonds. But that doesn't mean fat is bad. It just has to be eaten in proportion to other foods. A conventional serving size of almonds is only ¼ cup, but will ¼ cup of almonds by itself be a satisfying snack? Not for me. However, balance the almonds with protein and carbohydrates, like Greek yogurt and blueberries, and you can enjoy a smaller portion size and get full from fat in a good way.

Some of my clients go overboard on fats by eating too much of the good stuff. I had one client, Gretchen, who was trying to eat for better skin. Every day, she ate many servings of almond butter, avocados, salmon, and walnuts, making fat a disproportionately large part of her daily diet. Her skin looked great, but she couldn't understand why she was getting a muffin top hanging over her jeans.

Another client was scared of fat. Tessa overate carbohydrates to compensate for a lack of fat in her diet. Her favorites were low-fat cookies and low-fat brownies (loaded with sugar!). Tessa was 15 pounds overweight, and when we added fat back into her diet and took out the fake desserts, she was amazed that she lost all 15 pounds in just 4 weeks!

Studies show that people who consume low-fat versions of regular foods tend to eat more calories, probably because they overeat the foods that don't quite satisfy. Remember, fat makes you feel satisfied, triggering your brain to recognize when you've had enough and can stop eating.

Balancing with 1:1:1

Protein, carbs, and fat are all necessary parts of the human diet. They keep your body working correctly, your muscles strong, your energy level high, and your skin and hair beautiful. They will keep your blood sugar stable and your brain sharp, and they are responsible for thousands of chemical reactions that happen inside the body.

So don't skimp on any category! Respect your body's needs and the power of good nutrition. The best way to lose excess weight, feel good, and get or stay healthy is to eat all three in balance, and the easiest way to do this is by employing the 1:1:1 eating strategy.

Now that you know so much about nutrition and the importance of balance, we're ready for the nuts and bolts of eating 1:1:1. The next chapter will show you exactly how to do it.

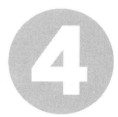

CHAPTER FOUR

The 411 on 1:1:1

When you sit down to talk to people about the path that brought them to weight gain and their experiences trying to drop those pounds, as I do several times a day, you hear a lot of stories. Of course, everyone is different and each journey is unique—on the surface. I've found, though, that when you go beyond the specific life circumstances, one factor is at the heart of everyone's weight woes: imbalance. The beauty of 1:1:1 is that it restores balance, even when your diet and your life *feel* out of balance. If you're not at a healthy weight, there's a reason. Are you ready to figure out what that is? Are you ready to get sane again? It's time to learn the 1:1:1 strategy, and put it into action—today. Eating according to 1:1:1 is simple, but you need to know some very important things before you can practice it effectively.

What Should You Eat?

Wait a minute, you might be thinking. *I thought she said she wasn't going to tell me what to eat!* You are correct! However, I will tell you how to balance your choices. This is the crux of the 1:1:1 plan, and it's practically self-explanatory. Every time you eat anything, it should consist of:

- 1 portion of protein
- 1 portion of carbohydrate
- 1 portion of fat

This is the primary and most important strategy. Even if you don't follow the other suggestions and guidelines I'll give you throughout the rest of this book, even if you never try 1:1:1 Accelerated (see Chapter 7), this strategy will still work. Because it naturally restricts calories without deprivation, it will ease your body back into balance painlessly. Remember, no food is off-limits, but never, ever skip one of your 1s. That means no carb-only snacks, no all-protein lunches, and no fat-free dinners. The days of ditching entire food categories, and the feeling of denial that accompanies that approach, are over for you.

Of course, you can't easily put together a meal with one portion each of protein, carb, and fat if you aren't totally sure which foods are primarily made of protein, which are mostly carbs, and which are considered fats. I'm always surprised how much my clients don't really know about the primary nutrient components of various foods. In case you're confused about this, too, you'll find lists of the foods that count as proteins, carbohydrates, and fats on pages 62–66. Whenever you're not sure, just check these lists.

Truthfully, most foods contain more than one of these macronutrients. For example, bread is a carb, but it does contain some protein, and often contains some fat, too. However, for our purposes, we are going with what the food item contains the *most* of. There are two exceptions, however.

About Double-Doers

A few foods are pretty evenly balanced between two macronutrient categories, and in those cases, you can count them as either one or the other. I call these foods "double-doers." For example, cheese contains protein and fat, so you can use it in a meal as either. With turkey and bread, it could be a fat. With apples and almonds, it could be a protein.

These foods are marked with superscripts in the lists starting on page 66, and they appear in more than one list. Cheese is in the protein list, with a superscript F, like this: cheese^F. This is to remind you that cheese is a protein, but it can also be a fat. On the fat list, cheese will have a superscript P, like this: cheese^P. This is to remind you that cheese is a fat, but it can also be a protein.

In practice, double-doers only increase your possibilities for meals. For instance, on a cheese pizza with vegetables, cheese could be the protein, leaving room for walnuts or avocado in your side salad. However, it could also be the fat, leaving room for pepperoni or sausage (protein) as an additional pizza topping. (Yes! You can have pepperoni pizza!)

Now let's think about beans. Beans are both a protein and a carb because they contain a high level of protein but also a lot of starch and fiber. In a bean burrito, they could count as a protein; the tortilla is the carb. In chili, however, beans can be the carb, when beef or turkey is the protein.

Chocolate is another example of a double-doer. Chocolate could be a fat or a carb. A few chocolate chips could be your fat on a waffle (carb), along with chicken-apple sausage for a protein. In Greek yogurt (protein), a few chocolate chips could be your carb, along with walnuts for the fat. Remember, double-doers will be listed in both categories to which they belong, but marked with a superscript to remind you which other category they could be applied to.

About Free Foods

Don't you love getting something for free? In the case of the 1:1:1 plan, nonstarchy vegetables and a few other foods are free! Although technically, all vegetables contain carbs, the nonstarchy kind (like leafy greens, broccoli, lettuce, and tomatoes) are so low in carbs and calories and so high in nutrients that I don't want you to feel you need to restrict them at all. When you're superhungry, this is where you can really go to town. Just keep the other foods in your meal in balance. The list on page 67 will tell you which foods are free.

1:1:1 Portion Sizes

But wait! There's something else extremely important to consider. Balance is crucial, but it's not the only factor. You're not going to lose weight eating a pound of pasta with a pound of meat sauce and a pound of cheese for dinner, even if that might look like 1:1:1 to you. To keep your body in proportion is to eat the right portions, and that's just too much food.

This is the other area where I see people getting into trouble, even when they're eating in balance. They overeat by choosing portions that are way too big, and they're so used to stuffing it in that they no longer notice when their bodies have had enough. However, you can get back to normal. It's time to reclaim your body's natural ability to feel full on a reasonable amount of food. When you choose one protein, one carb, and one fat, you are actually choosing one *portion* of protein, one *portion* of carbs, and one *portion* of fat. We all know, if we're totally honest with ourselves, that a pound of spaghetti is *not* a portion. It's more like eight portions. Portion sizes aren't really that complicated, and once you learn them and measure them out a few times, you can totally eyeball them. (But watch out for "portion creep"—that tendency to make portions subtly larger and larger until that 1 cup of pasta is back to 2 or 3 cups again.)

Most of the time, the portion size is obvious because it's listed on a food's package. But what about when the food isn't in a package? Maybe you got your brown rice from the bulk bin in the health food aisle, or you threw away the package and stored the food in a more airtight container (a good idea with cereal and snack foods), or the package doesn't state a serving size (as with, perhaps, a tray of chicken breasts from the meat counter)?

That's why I listed the recommended portion sizes on our protein, carb, and fat master lists. Use them to plan your breakfasts, lunches, and dinners (for snacks, see below) Don't fret—these portions are generous, not skimpy, but also not excessive. They're enough to fill up anyone who gets used to eating normal portion sizes again. Since you only get one protein, one carb, and one fat, you need to have enough of each—but not too much of any. This is how you'll know, for example, to eat a turkey and cheese sandwich made with two slices of bread (no more open-faced diet-y sandwiches, hooray!), 4 to 6 ounces of turkey deli meat (not 2 ounces, not 8 ounces), 1 ounce of cheese (not three slices, but hooray, you get cheese!), and of course, all the free veggies you want. This is plenty of food for anyone for a good lunch. Add club soda or water and go wild with the free vegetables—lettuce, tomato, sprouts, green peppers, etc. Knock yourself out! That's how you will make the meal truly filling, as well as give the nutritional content a significant bump. Isn't portion control awesome?

A Special Note About Snacks

The only difference between a 1:1:1 meal and a 1:1:1 snack is that meat and grain foods are cut to half portions. The purpose of this is to keep snacks from being the size of full meals. For example, a serving of turkey is 4 to 6 ounces, but if you are having deli turkey slices for a snack, you would cut back to 2 or 3 ounces. For grains, it's the same. If you have a bowl of cereal for a snack, you would cut your portion to ½ cup, instead of a full 1-cup serving. If you have crackers or chips, cut those portions to ½ ounce instead of a full ounce, as you would have for a regular meal. A sandwich becomes half a sandwich, using only 1 slice of bread. Other foods stay the same, however, so your snacks remain filling and nutritious. You can still have a full piece or cup of fruit, a full ounce of cheese, a full cup of cottage cheese, and, of course, all the free veggies you like.

The Lists

Now, on to what qualifies as a protein, constitutes a carb, and counts as a fat along with the recommended portion sizes for each food. These are your master lists, so refer to them whenever you need to check what a sweet potato counts as (carb), or whether quinoa is a double-doer (it is—carb and protein), or which foods are totally free (like zucchini!).

You may notice that some of these portions sizes are different from the ones listed on the package. That's okay! These are the portions for 1:1:1 that will maximize your satiety while ensuring your weight loss. You don't have to get obsessive about these portion sizes if you are in a restaurant or some other social situation, or are preparing a recipe. Just be sure you have approximately 1 protein, 1 carb, and 1 fat. When assembling your own meals and snacks, however, this is your portion size guide.

1:1:1 PROTEIN LIST

Every meal and snack must have a portion of protein. Now you know how important protein is for building muscle, repairing your body after exercise, and more, so don't skip it! Protein will also ease your hunger later, keeping your satiety level high. These are the foods that count as proteins on the 1:1:1 plan.

- Bacon[F] (all types, including bacon made from pork, turkey, or even salmon), *2 strips*
- Beans[C] and peas[C] (legumes), including lentils, black beans, white beans, pinto beans, chickpeas, dal, split peas, green peas, and black-eyed peas, *1 cup*
- Beef (steak, ground beef, roasts, hamburger, etc.), *4 to 6 ounces*
- Buffalo/bison (in all forms, steaks and ground), *4 to 6 ounces*

- Cheese[F] such as Swiss, American, Cheddar, provolone, mozzarella, goat cheese, feta, brie, blue cheese, string cheese, *1 ounce*
- Cream cheese[F], *1 ounce*
- Cottage cheese, *1 cup* (low-fat or fat-free is preferable)
- Deli meat, *4 to 6 ounces*
- Egg whites, *2*
- Eggs, whole[F], *1*
- Fish (fresh, frozen, or canned and raw or cooked, including salmon, tuna, halibut, trout, tilapia, cod, bass, sole), *4 to 6 ounces*

- Hummus^{C,F}, *½ cup*
- Jerky (made from any meat, poultry, or seafood), *1 ounce*
- Lamb (ground, loin, leg of lamb, shanks, etc.), *4 to 6 ounces*
- Milk and all milk products (whole, 2%, 1%, fat-free, and flavored milk), *1 cup*
- Pork (including pork chops, roasts, and ham), *4 to 6 ounces*
- Poultry (chicken, turkey, duck, Cornish game hen, etc.), *4 to 6 ounces*
- Protein bars, *1 (7 to 15 grams protein)*
- Protein powder (from whey, soy, rice, pea, or other protein sources), *1 scoop (between 10 and 20 grams protein)*
- Quinoa^C, *1 cup* cooked
- Ricotta cheese, *1 cup*

- Sausage, *3 ounces*
- Shellfish (lobster, shrimp, scallops, mussels, prawns, crayfish, etc.), *4 to 6 ounces*
- Soy milk, *1 cup*
- Soy yogurt, *¾ to 1 cup*
- Soy products, including edamame, tofu, tempeh, and soy-based imitation meat products like veggie burgers and veggie hot dogs, *4 to 6 ounces*
- Veal, *4 to 6 ounces*
- Wheat gluten and products made from it, including many imitation meat products such as fake shredded "chicken" and veggie hot dogs, *4 to 6 ounces*
- Yogurt (preferably Greek because it contains the most protein), *¾ to 1 cup*

1:1:1 CARB LIST

For most people, this is the toughest category to keep to a single portion. We love our comforting carbs, and we get to have them! It's just a matter of choosing which one you want for any given meal or snack (if this seems hard at first, just remind yourself that you've got another meal or snack coming in just a few hours—you can do it!). Cutting carbs to one portion per meal and snack is what will really speed up your weight loss. Choose from these options.

- Bagels, *1*
- Baked goods and pastries (muffins, cake, croissants, doughnuts, cupcakes, scones, etc.), *1*
- Barley, *1 cup cooked*
- Beans[P] (legumes) and peas[P], including lentils, black beans, white beans, pinto beans, chickpeas, dal, split peas, green peas, and black-eyed peas, *1 cup*
- Beer, *12 ounces*
- Biscuits, *1*
- Bread, *1 slice, unless having a sandwich, in which case have 2 slices*
- Bulgur, *1 cup cooked*
- Candy, *2 ounces*
- Chocolate[F], *1 tablespoon or 1 square*
- Chocolate-covered seeds or nuts[F], *1 tablespoon*
- Cocktail, *1½ ounce (1 shot) liquor, 1*
- Cold cereal, *1 cup*
- Cookies, *1 regular size or 3 small (or check package for serving size)*
- Corn, *1 ear or 1 cup kernels*
- Corn chips, *1 ounce*
- Corn tortillas, *2 small*
- Cornbread, *3-inch square*
- Couscous, *1 cup cooked*
- Crackers, *1 ounce*
- Cream of Wheat, *1 cup*
- Dinner rolls, *1*
- Dried fruit, such as raisins, prunes, cherries, *¼ cup*
- English muffins, *1*
- Flour tortillas, *1*
- French fries[F] (if baked, this is a carb only), *12 fries*
- Fruit, such as apples, medium bananas, strawberries, blueberries, raspberries, peaches, grapes, cherries, plums, oranges, nectarines, melons, pomegranates, papayas, mangos, pineapple, kiwifruits, coconut[F], *1 piece or 1 cup chopped fruit or berries*
- Graham crackers, *2 sheets*
- Granola, *⅓ cup*
- Grits, *1 cup cooked*
- Hamburger and hot dog buns, *1*

- Hummus[P, F], *½ cup*
- Ice cream, *½ cup*
- Matzoh, *1 sheet*
- Millet, *1 cup cooked*
- Oatmeal, *1 cup cooked*
- Pancakes, *1 medium (or 2 to 3 small)*
- Pasta, *1 cup cooked*
- Pitas, *1*
- Popcorn, *3 cups popped*
- Potato chips[F], *1 ounce*
- Potatoes, any type (white, blue, yellow, red, white), prepared any way (mashed, baked, shredded, fried, etc.), *1 medium or 1 cup*
- Pretzels, *1 ounce*
- Quinoa[P], *1 cup cooked*
- Rice, *1 cup cooked*
- Rice cereal, hot, *1 cup cooked*
- Sweetened nondairy creamer[F], *1 tablespoon*
- Sweeteners: cane sugar, honey, molasses, brown rice syrup, sorghum, maple syrup, corn syrup, jam, jelly, and preserves, *1 teaspoon*
- Sweet potatoes or yams, *1 medium or 1 cup*
- Sweet potato fries[F] (if baked, this a carb only), *12 fries*
- Taco shells, *1*
- Toaster pastries, *1*
- Waffles, *1*
- Wine, *4 ounces*
- Winter squashes such as acorn and butternut, *1 cup*

Food for **Thought**

People seem to be very confused by fruit. I'm not sure why. It's nature's candy, the perfect way to enjoy something sweet along with fiber and vitamins. I once had a client who loved bananas, but she thought they were bad for her, a guilty pleasure! Fruit is an excellent addition to your 1:1:1 meal, but it does count as a carb, and you only get one carb per meal. I had another client who was borderline diabetic. He told me he was eating five apples and a pound of grapes every day because he wanted to be healthy. We added it up: He was eating almost 1,000 calories per day in fruit alone! More of a good thing does not make it a better thing, but fruit *is* a good thing. Just keep it in balance.

1:1:1 FAT LIST

Fats also add to your feeling of satiety so you don't need to nosh constantly. Be sure every meal and snack has a portion. Choose from these fats.

- Avocado, *¼ medium*
- Bacon[P], *2 strips*
- Butter, *1 tablespoon*
- Chocolate[C], *1 tablespoon or 1 square*
- Chocolate-covered seeds or nuts[C], *1 tablespoon*
- Coconut (shredded) *1 tablespoon*
- Coconut milk, carton, *1 cup*
- Coconut milk, canned, *¼ cup*
- Cream, including whipped cream, *1 tablespoon*
- Eggs, whole[P], *1*
- Fried foods (such as french fries[C]), *12 small pieces or equivalent*
- Ghee (clarified butter), *1 tablespoon*
- Half-and-half, *1 tablespoon*

- Hummus[C,P], *½ cup*
- Mayonnaise, *1 tablespoon*
- Nondairy creamer (sweetened versions are double-doers also in the carb category, and fat-free versions are carb only), *1 tablespoon*
- Nut and seed butters, *1 tablespoon*
- Nuts and seeds, *1 tablespoon*
- Olives, *10 small or 5 large*
- Salad dressing (doesn't count on salad), *1 tablespoon*
- Sour cream, *1 tablespoon*
- Vegetable oils, including olive, canola, coconut, corn, soybean, and all-purpose vegetable oil (doesn't count if sautéing veggies), *1 tablespoon*

1:1:1 FREE FOODS LIST

You can *always* add any of the items on this list for free, if you so desire. When it comes to 1:1:1, these foods are invisible. They are a zero. They also happen to be superhealthy, but that doesn't mean you have to shove them in if you're not in the mood. These foods are a bonus, and a great addition to your diet. They also contain fiber, so they will help keep you full. However, they're also totally optional (although you may find that as you lose weight and feel better, these foods seem more and more appealing):

- Asparagus
- Beets
- Bell peppers
- Bok choy
- Broccoli
- Cabbage
- Carrots
- Cauliflower
- Celery
- Cucumber
- Dried spices and spice mixtures (like ground red pepper, cinnamon, black pepper, cumin, and sumac)
- Eggplant
- Extracts, all natural, like vanilla, peppermint, almond, etc.
- Fresh and dried herbs (like basil, oregano, thyme, cilantro, and parsley)
- Garlic
- Greens, both cooking greens (such as beet greens, collards, kale, mustard greens, Swiss chard) and salad greens (romaine lettuce, Bibb lettuce, arugula, spinach, spring mix, mesclun, microgreens, mache)
- Green beans
- Herbal tea
- Hot chile peppers (like jalapeños and poblanos)
- Hot sauce
- Leeks
- Lettuce (romaine, butter, red—see also Greens above)
- Onions
- Rutabagas
- Salsa
- Scallions
- Shallots
- Sprouts
- Summer squash
- Tomatoes, all types and colors, fresh and canned
- Tomato sauce
- Turnips
- Water, plain or sparkling
- Zucchini

How It All Adds Up

To help you see how all these food categories fit together—and how easy it is to follow—let's look at some real-world meal ideas. Remember, these are not meal plans you have to follow. They're only ideas to inspire you and demonstrate how the 1:1:1 plan will keep you in balance.

Breakfast

- A bowl of oatmeal (carb) with milk (protein) and walnuts (fat)
- Greek yogurt (protein) with almonds (fat) and blueberries (carb)
- Scrambled eggs (protein) with cheese (fat) and toast (carbohydrate)
- Leftovers from dinner the night before: steak (protein) with mashed potatoes (carb) and butter (fat)
- Cold pepperoni pizza (crust is the carb, pepperoni is the protein, cheese is the fat)

Do you see how flexible 1:1:1 can be? Sure, leftover pizza isn't the best breakfast choice, and as a nutritionist, I'd steer you toward one of the first three options because they're more nutritious. But if you wake up one morning and you just really, really want cold pizza, then you can still have it without feeling like you "ruined" anything.

Midmorning Snack

- Hummus (protein) with a drizzle of olive oil (fat) and pita wedges (carb). Add mixed vegetables (free) to make it more filling and nutritious, if you like.
- Apple slices (carb), half topped with cheese (protein) and half spread with almond butter (fat)
- Whole grain cereal (carb) with milk (protein) and a few walnuts (fat)
- A mini whole wheat pita (carb) with hummus (fat) and pastrami (protein)

Anything goes for your snack, as long as it's balanced. Yes, even candy! (Just try not to have candy *every* day, and keep it to a single serving, as listed on the package.)

Lunch

- A roast chicken (protein) sandwich on a hard roll (carb) with avocado (fat), and tomato (free)

- A big salad topped with chicken (protein), strawberries (carb), walnuts (fat), and veggies (free). Dressing goes with the salad.

- A scoop of tuna salad (protein plus fat from the mayonnaise) with whole-grain crackers (carb)

- Chili made with ground beef (protein) and beans (carb) and garnished with sour cream (fat)

- Chicken (protein) noodle (carbohydrate) soup full of vegetables (free), with crackers (carb)

- Corn chowder made with corn (carb), black beans (protein), and heavy cream (fat)

Sounds great, right? I bet by now you can think of a hundred more options.

Midafternoon Snack

- Dried apricots (carb) with a cheese stick (protein) and almonds (fat)

- Cottage cheese (protein) topped with blueberries (carb) and chopped hazelnuts (fat)

- Whole grain toast (carb) with roast beef (protein) and Swiss cheese (fat)

- Strawberries (carb) dipped in ricotta cheese (protein) and dark chocolate (fat)

Yep, you can have chocolate! Just balance it according to 1:1:1.

Dinner

- Steak (protein) with a baked potato or rice (carbohydrate) and butter or sour cream (fat)

- Pasta (carb) with shrimp (protein) and a sprinkle of Parmesan cheese (fat)

- Grilled chicken (protein) salad full of greens and sliced vegetables (free). Save your carb and fat for dessert, such as a bowl of fresh berries (carb) drizzled with heavy cream or a dollop of whipped cream (fat). Or have bread (carb) with your salad and a piece of dark chocolate (fat) for dessert.

- Salmon steak (protein), asparagus (free) topped with Hollandaise sauce (fat), and a glass of wine (carb)

- A hearty stew made with lamb (protein), sweet potatoes (carb), and lots of chunky vegetables (free), with a side salad (free) topped with avocado (fat)

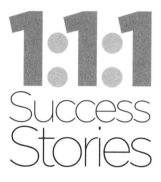

1:1:1 Success Stories

Name: **Mikaal Shoaib**
Starting weight: **230 pounds**
Current weight: **200 pounds**
Height: **6'**

I always thought I was healthy. I really didn't know much about food, but I worked out with a trainer and ate what he recommended— mostly protein shakes and nutrition bars, although I did not particularly like the taste of either.

Then I moved across the country for work and stopped exercising for a while. When I finally joined a gym, I made an appointment to meet with a trainer. He took some basic body measurements— height, weight, blood pressure, etc. I was shocked to discover that I weighed 230 pounds and my blood pressure was high enough that the club required me to get a physician's authorization before I could work out with the trainer. That was when I realized I needed to do something about my overall fitness and well-being, including my diet.

How Often Should You Eat?

I spend a lot of time advising my clients about the *timing* of their meals There's a lot of confusion out there. People have heard that it's healthy to graze all day long, but they don't understand the meaning of *graze*. It certainly does not mean eating full-size meals many times a day. Then there are people in the "snacking is bad" camp. They don't realize that when you stick to three meals, chances are those meals will be huge because you'll be starving every time you sit down to eat. Ditto for the breakfast and lunch skippers. It's surprising how deeply rooted people's

I decided to see the club's nutritionist, and it turned out to be Rania. She asked what my goals were, but I didn't know! All I knew was that I wanted to improve my overall health and lose some weight. I mentioned that I had a high-stress job (I'm a lawyer at a large firm) and therefore didn't have time to grocery shop and cook meals for myself. In fact, I hadn't turned on the oven in my apartment since I'd moved in several months earlier.

Rania introduced me to 1:1:1 and showed me how the strategy could fit with my life. Soon, I was eating balanced meals for the first time. And the strategy held up even when I had to attend business lunches and dinners, ate at restaurants with friends, or was on vacation. I became more thoughtful about the food I was consuming. And although I was eating smaller portions, I never felt hungry.

I began to feel that my body was working efficiently, as it was intended to. I'd often get up at 5:30 a.m. to go to the health club, but I wouldn't be tired. On the 1:1:1 plan, I lost 30 pounds in 4 months. I'm at a healthy weight for my height and build, and I have a lifestyle I can stick with no matter how crazy my life gets!

111

Start-Now Strategy

Most people don't eat enough vegetables, and most are too narrow in their vegetable choices, sticking to only the three or four types they've had before (typically lettuce, tomato, carrots, and celery). Believe it or not, there are hundreds of delicious and amazing vegetables out there to choose from. Why limit yourself? Vegetables are your best opportunity for nutrient-dense eating. They're low in calories and have tons of vitamins, minerals, antioxidants, and fiber. You can always add vegetables to a meal and they'll only make your meal more nutritious.

Once, I asked a client what vegetables he ate. He told me he only ate vegetables when he was dieting.

"Why?" I asked him. I'd literally never heard anyone say this.

"Because they're diet food," he said.

There are a lot of diet foods that I don't consider real foods, but vegetables are certainly not on that list!

---

preferred patterns are: The grazers don't want to give up the "freedom" to eat all day long, and the anti-snackers and meal skippers are afraid if they veer from their habits their bodies will balloon. Truth is, even if every meal and snack was perfectly balanced according to 1:1:1, both of these eating patterns make it very difficult to lose weight. That's why I make it a point to help my clients find balance, not just in the composition of their meals and snacks, but in their timing.

Over the years, I've discovered that there is an optimal number of times to eat per day, and I've made this part of the 1:1:1 plan. That number is five, broken down into breakfast, midmorning snack, lunch, midafternoon snack, and dinner.

On this eating schedule, you'll stay satisfied, so you don't overeat at meals or have too many snacks. Eating five times per day puts your body back into balance and keeps your blood sugar level and on an even keel. This will keep you from experiencing surges of uncontrollable hunger when your blood sugar goes too low.

Note that there is no evening snack. *This is very important!* Don't think this is a misprint and you'd better add a snack to enjoy while you catch up on your TV shows. I don't want you eating anything after dinner because the body performs many tasks essential to healthy weight loss while you sleep, including tissue repair and toxin removal. This takes energy, but you've already got plenty of energy for these jobs in your own fat stores. You don't need to be wasting your body's precious healing resources on digestion. What's more, you don't need an influx of calories right before you're about to lie unconscious for 8 hours. That evening snack is more likely to get converted to fat because it will likely contain more calories than you need while sleeping. That's not to say your body doesn't use energy (in other words, burn calories) while you sleep. It does, for healing and dreaming and all kinds of biochemical processes. If you don't have an evening snack, guess where your body will get that energy? That's right: from your fat stores, which is exactly what you want if you're trying to drop pounds.

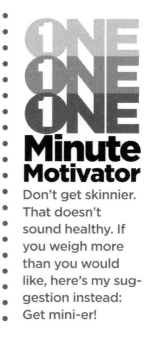

One One One Minute Motivator

Don't get skinnier. That doesn't sound healthy. If you weigh more than you would like, here's my suggestion instead: Get mini-er!

Although some studies say it doesn't matter when you eat, I disagree. Other studies support my view. One study reported in the *American Journal of Physiology* involved 11 healthy women in their twenties, who consumed an approximately 200-calorie snack at either 10 a.m. or 11 p.m. Compared to the daytime snackers, the nighttime snackers showed significantly less fat burning and a significantly increased level of total and LDL ("bad") cholesterol, suggesting that nighttime snacking negatively impacts fat metabolism and could increase the risk of obesity.

Nighttime eating is also more likely to cause digestive upset, including acid reflux. You're likely to sleep better and feel more comfortable if you go to sleep with your dinner fully digested, and nothing else rattling around in your stomach. A Brazilian study of 27 women and 25 men showed a correlation between late-night snacks and impaired sleep quality.

Fortunately, nighttime eating is usually just a bad habit. The next time you're tempted to eat at night, think about whether you'd rather be storing the fat from that half a bag of potato chips while you sleep or burning off some thigh jiggle.

Do you see how easy this is? One protein, one carb, one fat, five times a day, to stay satiated. Then pay attention to how you feel when you eat. If it's too much food, don't finish it. You'll get to eat again soon.

And there you have it—everything you need to know to get started *stat*.

Maybe you still have questions, and I bet you do, because as simple as it sounds, 1:1:1 can seem complicated when you start practicing it in the real world. Never fear—I'll answer all your how-to questions in Chapter 8. But first, I want to show you some food logs and help you start your own, so you can see just how close—or how far—you are from living 1:1:1 right now.

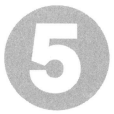

CHAPTER FIVE

Food Diaries: Diagnosing Your Diet

H ere's a truth: Clients don't always tell me the truth. It's not malicious and sometimes they aren't even aware that they aren't telling the truth. But when it comes to knowing, remembering, or admitting the amounts and types of foods they eat, people tend to err on the "angelic" side. I hear things like, "I really do eat a lot of vegetables" and "I hardly ever eat sugar" and "I know I only eat about 1,200 calories a day."

Uh-huh.

As a nutritionist, I know two things: Except in the case of an unusual medical problem, it's impossible to eat a healthy, balanced, calorie-restricted diet consistently and *not* lose excess weight. I don't care what you've heard about how someone who weighs 300 pounds may actually eat less than someone who weighs 150 pounds. Sure, maybe now and then, or on a particular day, this could be true, but over the long haul, no.

People either truly believe or fool themselves into believing that they're eating less than they really are. This isn't just my opinion. Studies show it. There are various ways to verify what people say they eat. In one study from the United Kingdom, which appeared in the journal *Cancer Epidemiology, Biomarkers and Prevention,* a group of obese volunteers filled out food diaries. According to the information they gave the researchers, they ate no more sugar than normal-weight participants. However, when their urine and blood were tested for sugar, the results suggested that the obese volunteers were clearly eating more than they indicated. Another study, discussed in the *Journal of the American Dietetic Association*, revealed that study participants underreported their calorie intake by as much as thousands of calories per day.

I don't believe these people lied on purpose. However, what I see in my practice reflects what the studies suggest, and when I press my clients to be totally honest, I begin to see what's really going on. A client might have a "good day" and then think that justifies 3 subsequent days of overeating—but why report those slipups to the nutritionist, who might judge her? Report the good day instead!

The truth is, your "good" days are not reflective of your total diet, and you may be having fewer of those "good" days than you think if you don't actually keep track.

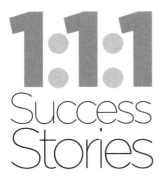

Success Stories

Name: **Bonnie Gothmann**
Starting weight: **150 pounds**
Current weight: **125 pounds**
Height: **5′6″**

I've always been athletic. I did 10K races, water aerobics, step classes, and worked out with a personal trainer so I could get in the weight training I wasn't doing on my own. I thought I was eating healthy and watching my fats, but I still wasn't losing the weight

Part of the problem is laxity. People just don't notice little things here and there. They forget about the supermarket samples or the leftover bites of the kids' meals or those two innocent spoonfuls of ice cream on the way to bed. They conveniently forget that cookie binge in front of the TV at night or that third slice of pizza, either because they just couldn't bring themselves to admit to it on paper or because they genuinely forgot about it. (It's often mindless eating, after all.) But it all counts, folks, and if you aren't paying attention, those little bits and bites can add up to a lot of calories and a lot of weight gain, as well as throw your entire diet out of balance.

So when clients tell me that they really don't eat very much, or eat plenty of vegetables, or rarely eat sugar, I don't exactly raise my eyebrows, but I do ask for proof. I ask them to keep a food diary, and to be as absolutely honest as they can. Every bite, every nibble counts. I promise not to judge them, only to teach them how to adjust things—and of course I can't make an honest assessment of anyone's problems if the food diary isn't accurate.

Keeping an accurate food diary can make a huge difference in the choices you make, as long as you're vigilant about reporting every

---

that I wanted to take off and keep off. I've always been a yo-yo dieter. I've been on all sorts of diets in my life. You name it and I've tried it. When I started working with Rania, however, she gave me a realistic plan I could stick with: 1:1:1! I began eating a variety of foods and the 1:1:1 concept was very easy for me to follow. I began to see my eating as a lifestyle choice rather than a diet. The results have been fantastic! I now feel a freedom around food that I never thought was possible. I know how to eat the correct food combinations at every meal and snack, and knowing that I can always switch it up without blowing it and that I always have choices has made all the difference in the world!

little thing—nothing goes into your mouth without getting written down! Studies confirm this works. Research from the Fred Hutchinson Cancer Research Center showed that among 123 overweight or obese sedentary women between the ages of 50 and 75, those who kept honest, complete food journals consistently lost about 6 pounds more than those who didn't keep track of what they ate. Of all the weight control strategies in the study (such as skipping meals), the strategy most associated with successful weight loss was keeping a food diary. Another study from Kaiser Permanente's Center for Health Research, one of the largest and longest-running weight loss maintenance trials ever conducted, found that keeping a food diary *doubled* weight loss.

I'd like you to take advantage of this fantastic weight loss tool. Even better, I'm going to teach you how I analyze the food diaries of my clients, so you can analyze your own, to see where *you* are out of balance.

Breaking It Down

I know. You're rolling your eyes, right? I can hear that deep, world-weary sighing. People hate to keep food diaries. They think they're too busy or it's too tedious. But are you too busy to be healthy? Is putting effort toward your future slim figure too tedious? Here's the thing: If your doctor told you to track your blood pressure so he could accurately diagnose a heart condition, or your fertility specialist told you to track your temperature so she could help you have a baby, you'd do it, wouldn't you?

Great. You know how to comply with instructions from a health professional that impact your health. Therefore, if your nutritionist tells you to keep a food diary, you should take it just as seriously. *And as your nutritionist, that's exactly what I'm telling you to do.* Your weight impacts everything about your health (including both your heart and your fertility!), so let's get this diagnosis correct.

A food diary is a peek into your eating habits. If you are totally, brutally honest, it can help you to see where you're going wrong and why.

I'd like to break down your food diary into two parts. First, keep track of what you typically eat for 3 days. This is hard because you'll want to be "good" for the food diary, and you're probably anxious to get started with 1:1:1, but this exercise will be more useful if you eat the way you normally would, pre-1:1:1. This is how you'll be able to analyze your habits and your normal way of eating. If you don't keep a food diary on a few "normal" days, you may not realize that you're overeating at lunch or undereating at breakfast or having too many snacks.

Next, I'll show you some sample food diaries from a few of my actual clients, along with my commentary about how they could easily tweak those meals to get them into balance using 1:1:1. And then, I want you to keep a food diary again, practicing 1:1:1—this time for the long haul, or at least until you get used to following 1:1:1 and don't feel the need to keep track anymore (but always go back to your food diary if you start to slip). This exercise will show you how you can eat the foods you love, the foods you *already eat,* and still lose weight doing it.

Okay, so let's start with you. Take 3 typical days out of your life, and record every bite you eat. I mean it! Every sip of mocha latte, every taste of ice cream, every cracker. Every cracker *crumb.* Put them all down. Don't

Food for **Thought**

Calorie counting takes time, even when you use those supposedly handy online trackers. When you can't find anything approximating what you eat, or the right brand, or you see multiple listings with widely varying calorie counts, it can be frustrating. Plus, some people get major anxiety when they see that fateful calorie number. Who has time for that? When you just write down what you eat, you can see how it flows over the course of your day and where you're going out of balance, without ever looking up a single calorie value. In fact, I believe worrying about calories is so overwhelming it may deter people from tracking what they eat. So forget calories! Just write down what you eat and work with that. It's all the information you need.

be afraid. I'm not asking you to count up the calories or show your food diary to anyone. Just write down the foods. You have to look your diet squarely in the eye if you actually want to fix what's not working. Remember, you're not practicing 1:1:1 for these 3 days. This is *You: Not on a Diet.*

There's a space on this chart for meals and snacks, but I'm definitely not saying you need to fill in every column. If you skip breakfast, leave it blank. If you don't have a midafternoon snack, leave it blank. If you eat late at night, admit it! Just eat the way you normally do, but *write it down.* Remember, this is just for you—the one person you should never, ever delude about what and how much you are eating.

	Breakfast	**Midmorning Snack**	**Lunch**	
Day 1:				
Day 2:				
Day 3:				

After you've filled out this chart (or made your own version in a notebook or on your computer or smartphone), take a good, hard look with a critical eye. Your imbalances may be obvious to you, but they may not. To help you get more practice analyzing food diaries (and to help you see some of the patterns you might be falling into), I've provided some sample pages from the food diaries of my clients (to protect their privacy, their names have been changed), along with my commentary to show you where they're going out of balance. See what they ate, read my comments, and then you can "play nutritionist" on your own food diary!

Midafternoon Snack	Dinner	Evening Snack

The Classic Carb Lover's Food Log

Maggie thinks she eats a healthy diet, and in many ways, she does. A 25-year-old waitress who sings in a band in the evenings, she knows she needs to look good for the stage. However, she doesn't understand why she can't seem to break through her weight loss plateau and get rid of

	Breakfast	Midmorning Snack	Lunch
Monday	1 packet instant organic maple syrup oatmeal + 1 mug Earl Grey tea *This meal needs a fat and a protein to help keep blood sugar stable. You could add 1 tablespoon walnuts (fat) and a cup of low-fat milk (protein), and you'll stay satisfied longer.*	1 banana + 1 mug Earl Grey tea *After an all-carb breakfast, you've chosen an all-carb snack. The banana is a healthy choice, but it's a carb choice and it needs balance. Make a smoothie with 1 banana, 1 cup coconut milk (the kind in the carton, not the can), and 1 tablespoon almond butter— and a dash of cinnamon for free! Add 1/2 cup ice and blend.*	Homemade chicken pasta with 3 cups pasta, 2 ounces chicken, 1/2 cup asparagus, 2 green olives *This fits the 1:1:1 formula, but the portions are out of whack. Take this down to 1 cup pasta. Increase the chicken to 4 to 6 ounces and increase the asparagus (or any combination of low-starch veggies) to 1 cup to reduce the calories and up the nutrition. The olives are your fat—but have more—about 10 small is a serving. You could also replace them with 1 tablespoon of grated Parmesan cheese if you like.*

those 15 extra pounds. As soon as I looked at Maggie's food diary, I could see the problem. She is a carb lover, and for many of her meals, she doesn't get any protein. Here is a Monday from Maggie's diary:

Midafternoon Snack	Dinner	Evening Snack
6 hazelnuts	At a restaurant: 1 sheet of lavash bread with herbs and feta cheese (appetizer) + 1 grilled salmon and bell pepper kebab + 1 cup basmati rice	None
Any kind of nut makes a satisfying, healthy snack and I suggest mixing them up because they're all slightly different nutritionally. But on their own they aren't balanced. Make a parfait—add a piece of fruit as a carb and add a Greek yogurt for protein.	*The lavash and the rice are both carbs, so pick one. You can always make a different choice next time.*	*Good! I generally discourage eating at night, and if your day of eating was truly balanced, you probably won't be hungry at night.*

The "I Thought This Was Diet Food" Food Log

My next client is a man I'll call John. John was a former athlete and was always a big eater, but now that he's hit 30 and doesn't work out as often, he's gained about 20 pounds. He came to me to help him take it

	Breakfast	Midmorning Snack	Lunch
Tuesday	2 whole wheat banana muffins with butter + ¼ cantaloupe + 2 turkey sausage links + 1 cup coffee with sugar *This breakfast is too heavy on the carbs. You've got 2 muffins and fruit. Bring this down to 1 muffin and save the fruit for your mid-morning snack. The butter on the muffin is fine. That's your fat. The turkey sausage is your protein, but remember, portion size matters. Sausage is 3 ounces.*	None *Here's where you can have the melon. Combine it with an ounce of turkey jerky and 1 tablespoon of cashews for a perfect 1:1:1 snack. You'll be more energized and less hungry at lunch.*	Tuna salad on whole wheat bread with mayo, pickle, and scallions + 1 slice leftover grilled pizza bianca with olive oil and Parmesan cheese + 1 apple *Sandwich or pizza— it's your choice, but to lose weight, save one or the other for a midafternoon snack. Both are complete 1:1:1 meals. The apple is another carb—save it for later.*

off. This is a Tuesday from his food diary. You may be able to tell that he was eating in a way he thought would help him lose weight. See where he got off track:

Midafternoon Snack	Dinner	Evening Snack
1 small bag baked chips	Broccoli pesto on bowtie pasta +	1 can light beer +
	boiled carrots with butter and dill +	3 cups popcorn
Baked chips are only a little better than regular chips and this isn't a balanced snack. Pair this with a string cheese for protein and dip the chips in a little bit of guacamole or hummus for fat.	raspberries and yogurt	*A carb-heavy, protein-deficient dinner probably led to evening hunger (unless it's just a habit). Balance your dinner according to 1:1:1 so it truly satisfies, and you won't need to snack at night.*
	Pasta is your carb and the pesto (made with nuts and olive oil) is your fat. You don't need butter on the carrots. Instead, steam them and toss them into the pasta. Also, watch your pasta portion sizes. Have just 1 cup. And where is your protein? Add some chicken–apple sausage to your pasta, and skip the yogurt and berries—you don't need them.	

The Meat Lover's Food Log

Adrian is a 35-year-old lawyer who loves his meat. He tried a low-carb diet for a while and enjoyed it, but eventually he missed his carbs. "Steak requires potatoes!" he told me. As so often happens, however, as soon as he went off his low-carb plan, he gained a lot of weight. He eats pretty

	Breakfast	Midmorning Snack	Lunch	
Wednesday	2 fried eggs + 2 strips bacon + 2 slices whole wheat toast with butter + 2 cups black coffee *This breakfast has more fat than what is ideal for weight loss. Take it down a notch with 1 egg and 1 slice of whole wheat toast. Keep the bacon but skip the butter—you won't miss the butter if you make an open-face sandwich and put the egg and bacon on top of the toast.*	None *Once we slim down your breakfast, you'll be ready for a mid-morning snack. A mid-morning snack will help you eat less at lunch. Have something simple you can take to the office with you, like an apple with a piece of string cheese and a few nuts.*	Philly cheesesteak sandwich + french fries + 1 diet soda *The sandwich is a 1:1:1 meal on its own, with the bun (carb), steak (protein), and cheese (fat). Skip the fries and have vegetables instead if you need more to fill you up.* *Consider swapping out the diet soda for water. It has no calories, but it can mess with your biochemistry, causing your body to expect calories without getting them, which can generate excessive hunger later.*	

well in general because he prefers home-cooked food, and he's lucky enough to be married to someone who loves to cook. However, he tends to overdo his portion sizes and sometimes he overeats carbs. Let's look at how his Wednesday went, after I counseled him about 1:1:1.

Midafternoon Snack	Dinner	Evening Snack
1 large handful peanuts	8-ounce sirloin steak +	10 whole wheat crackers with 10 small slices of cheese +
	1 cup mashed potatoes +	
	1 cup green beans +	1 diet soda
Your handful may be different than mine! Check the portion list and combine those nuts with some dried fruit and a few chocolate chips for a 1:1:1-appropriate snack.	1 glass red wine	
	Close! But choose one of your carbs—either the potatoes or the wine. For fat, go with a dollop of butter on your green beans or a spoonful of sour cream on those mashed potatoes to add fat.	*If you snack consistenly during the day, you won't need to snack at night, when you don't need those extra calories. Also, the caffeine in the soda will disrupt your sleep. Try a cup of herbal or decaf tea or some sparkling water with lime.*

The Rule Lover's Food Log

Maryam is a 26-year-old high school teacher and one of those chronic dieters who likes to have rules in place and be told exactly what to eat. Whenever she went off a diet, she'd gain all her weight back because she didn't have any rules to follow. When she first came to see me, she was 25 pounds over her goal weight. At first, she found 1:1:1 to be almost too freeing. "It's not strict enough!" she said. "Well, no," I said. "It's not strict, but it works."

	Breakfast	Midmorning Snack	Lunch
Thursday	1 cup oatmeal with blueberries, brown sugar, and skim milk + coffee with fat-free milk *Instead of having double carbs (oatmeal and blueberries), save the blueberries for your midmorning snack and add 1 tablespoon chopped walnuts and a sprinkle of cinnamon to your oatmeal for the sweet experience without the sugar.*	None *Now is your chance to have those blueberries. Pair them up with 1 cup Greek yogurt or cottage cheese for protein. Sprinkle in some sliced almonds if you like them, or even a teaspoon of mini chocolate chips for some fat.*	White bean soup with summer squash + arugula salad + ½ mango + 1 chocolate chip cookie *The vegetables will help fill you up while the beans provide protein. Add a fat, such as parmesan, to the arugula salad. Choose either the mango or the cookie as your carb; make the other part of your afternoon snack.*

Maryam wanted a meal plan, but I encouraged her to get back in touch with her own tastes, preferences, and hunger so she could finally be free from dieting, and she's making great progress. This is an example of a Thursday for Maryam. You'll see she's doing a pretty good job sticking to 1:1:1 and only needs the occasional tweak to her choices.

Midafternoon Snack	Dinner	Evening Snack
½ peanut butter sandwich on whole wheat bread + 1 cup fat-free milk *Well done! You skipped the jam on the sandwich and added in protein with the fat-free milk. It's a perfect 1:1:1 snack.*	Baked shrimp with feta cheese, tomatoes, onions, garlic, herbs and 1 tablespoon olive oil + salad with red wine vinaigrette + 1 pita + 1 banana *It's OK to cook your veggies with a little olive oil and have salad dressing. However, you've got an extra carb in there. Choose either the pita or the banana, but not both.*	None *Good job today! Keep tweaking to stay in line with 1:1:1 and your weight will keep going down.*

The Junk Food Junkie's Food Log

Tom is a 27-year-old, self-proclaimed junk food addict who even argued with me that he should still be able to eat it, until he realized that I wasn't arguing back! So-called junk food can be fine once in a while, as long as

	Breakfast	Midmorning Snack	Lunch
Friday	At a diner: 1 bowl strawberries + 1 cup roasted potatoes + cheese omelet + 1 slice sourdough toast with butter and jam *There are simply too many carb choices here. Pick either the strawberries, sourdough toast, or potatoes. Have 2 eggs, not 3. If you choose the bread, skip the jam and butter. You could also have (free) mushrooms, bell peppers, and onions with the omelet if you need more.*	1 ham sandwich with mayo, lettuce, tomato, and Swiss cheese + 1 plum + 1 cup V-8 juice *This looks more like a meal than a snack. Cut back to 1 slice of bread with 1 ounce of Swiss cheese and 3 ounces of ham. V-8 is fine (it's free), but sliced veggies may be more satisfying. Skip the plum for now and save it for your mid-afternoon snack.*	2 slices veggie pizza with mozzarella cheese + 1 large salad with honey-mustard dressing + fresh pineapple slices + 1 small handful chocolate-covered almonds *There are a lot of carbs and fats in this meal. Save the almonds and the pineapple for a snack. Have one slice of veggie pizza (carbs + fat) and add protein, like chicken, to the pizza, or beans to the salad.*

you balance it according to 1:1:1. Tom, however, often neglected this balancing act, and the extra 40 pounds he was carrying proved it. This is an example of a Friday before he started the 1:1:1 plan in earnest.

Midafternoon Snack	Dinner	Evening Snack
None	At a drive-thru:	Chocolate-almond candy bar
	2 cheeseburgers +	
A mid-afternoon snack can be more critical than a mid-morning snack because the time between lunch and dinner is often several hours. Looking at your dinner today, I suspect you were pretty hungry on your way home. Better to snack when you first start to get hungry than to wait for a late dinner and then overdo it. Enjoy 1 tablespoon of those dark chocolate-covered almonds (fat) now, with the pineapple slices (carb) and Greek yogurt (protein).	1 small order fries +	
	1 diet soda +	*I'm guessing that all those carbs in the drive-thru left you even hungrier. Also, eating in the car likely left you feeling deprived because you never sat down for a real dinner. Instead, do dinner right and you won't need candy before bed.*
	apple pie	
	(ate it in the car on the way home)	
	This is what happens when you wait too long for dinner without snacking! However, you can still go through the drive-thru. You have 3 carbs here—the bread on both your burgers, the fries, and the apple pie. If you want a burger, work with 1:1:1. Get a larger burger with cheese for a 1:1:1 meal. If you want either the fries or the apple pie, then you need to pick a salad for dinner with some protein, like chicken or a bowl of chili. You have to make a choice here.	

The Rockin' 1:1:1 Food Log

The last food diary I want to show you belongs to Alice. Alice is a 42-year-old mother of a teenager who is finally making herself a priority after realizing she was almost 30 pounds overweight. She's being practicing the 1:1:1

	Breakfast	Midmorning Snack	Lunch	
Saturday	1 whole egg scrambled with spinach, tomatoes, and onions + 1 slice toasted Ezekiel bread with almond butter	6 ounces nonfat vanilla bean Greek yogurt + ½ cup pomegranate seeds + 1 tablespoon crushed walnuts	1 grilled cheese and tomato sandwich on Ezekiel bread + 1 cup roasted squash with olive oil	
	This is a great breakfast. Eggs (protein), sprouted grain toast (carb), and almond butter (fat) make the perfect balance, and of course, all those nutritious veggies are free.	*Great job! The pomegranate seeds contain fiber and nutrients and serve as your carb. The yogurt is your protein and the walnuts are your fat.*	*Another perfect 1:1:1 meal. Grilled cheese is so satisfying. Great job pairing it up with the roasted squash flavored with olive oil for a little fat.*	

Now it's *your* turn. You've done your initial 3 days, so look back. After seeing what I wrote on the food diaries of my clients, what do you think I would write on *your* food diary? Channel your inner nutritionist and be critical. Where are you going out of balance? How many protein, carb, and fat servings are you eating at each meal? How could you trim them down to 1:1:1?

When I have my clients try this for themselves, they find it extremely enlightening. It helps them to look at what they're doing in a more objective way. Suddenly, they realize they need to take responsibility for everything that goes into their mouths, and they also feel empowered because they realize that they know exactly what they should be doing.

Once you've examined your food log with a more practiced eye, I'd like strategy for almost 2 months, and she's already lost 18 pounds. You'll see below what good choices she makes! I'm so proud of her. This is her typical Saturday. Notice how she works in comfort food while staying in balance.

Midafternoon Snack	Dinner	Evening Snack
1 pumpkin muffin with butter +	6-ounce panko-crusted tilapia +	None
1 glass fat-free milk	1 cup green beans with 1 tablespoon slivered almonds +	*You'll be burning fat all night long! Keep up the good work.*
This is a fine snack. The muffin is a carb, the milk is a protein, and the butter is your fat.	1 glass of wine	
	I like this meal a lot. The fish is the protein, and the slivered almonds sprinkled over the green beans are the fat. Wine is your carb.	

you to try keeping one for a whole week—but this time, do it while you are practicing 1:1:1. At the end of each day, take a good, hard look at it the way I would. Were you successful? Where did you slip up, and why? Did you skip a snack? Go too heavy on the carbs or skip the fat? Keep making your own commentary, just as you did before you started practicing 1:1:1.

Are you ready? It's time to start practicing! You are a 1:1:1 eater now. As you go through your day making your meal and snack choices, write in the chart on the next page, what you eat then make your commentary at the end of the day. Note how well you did and how you might fix things to be more in balance at the next meal. Make a copy of the chart, or fill it out right here in the book. Of course, you can also do this on your computer or phone. Now get to the diagnosis! (And don't forget to enjoy your food.)

My 1:1:1 Diary

	Breakfast	Midmorning Snack	
Day 1			
YOUR ANALYSIS:			
Day 2			
YOUR ANALYSIS:			
Day 3			
YOUR ANALYSIS:			

Lunch	Midafternoon Snack	Dinner

CHAPTER SIX

Meal Plans and Snack Ideas

bet you're ready to get down to business and start eating, right? Go ahead! You don't need anyone's permission, and you don't need a meal plan to enjoy a delicious 1:1:1 meal. In fact, you can totally skip this chapter if you like—or read it purely for inspiration.

One of the most popular aspects of the 1:1:1 plan is that you can eat anything, anywhere. You can go out to eat or for drinks, eat with friends, or do anything else you want to do. You're free! Just remind yourself to follow the 1:1:1 strategy before you put something in your mouth, balance accordingly, and you're good to go.

However, some of my clients like more guidance. They want a meal plan. I sit down with them and we go over their food diary and talk about the foods they like to eat. Then I show them exactly how they can still have their favorites and lose weight. Maybe you'd like that, too. That's why I've put together a full week of real meals made with real food, every one of them balanced according to 1:1:1. I can't customize it to your individual preferences, but *you* can. Don't like chicken? Sub in beef. Don't like salmon? Swap it for chicken. Don't like rice? Have pasta instead. Don't eat cheese? Try a drizzle of olive oil or some avocado. There are a million ways to make these meal plans *yours*. I only include them here to help you begin putting meals together.

I've come up with a week's worth of meals—seven breakfasts, seven lunches, seven dinners, and seven snacks—for you to choose from, play with, alter, or ignore completely. You'll see how each meal works because I've listed the components according to the category they fall into—protein, carbohydrate, or fat. I also list free foods you can have with your balanced meal, with special instructions on how to combine everything to make a delicious 1:1:1 meal or why a recipe is already a complete 1:1:1 meal in itself. After 7 days, you're going to be a pro.

Remember, this is not a *required* meal plan! The only rule is 1:1:1, so if you want to swap out any item in any meal in exchange for another equal item (say, to trade tofu for a chicken breast, a bagel for an English muffin, or even a piece of fruit for a doughnut), go for it. It's your meal, it's your food, it's your life, and it's your 1:1:1.

For more inspiration, turn to the recipes at the back of this book. I've provided 75 of them to get you started with lots of ideas for 1:1:1 meals and snacks. When an item in the meal plan is a recipe in the back, I've given you the page number.

Seven 1:1:1 Breakfasts

They say breakfast is the most important meal of the day, but that doesn't mean you have to limit yourself to breakfast-y foods. It can be about eggs and bacon or waffles and syrup if you like, but it can also be something crazy like cold spaghetti with meatballs or leftover pizza or pita with hummus and raw vegetables! It all depends on what you want. Here are some conventional breakfast meals for you to try, but don't feel held back by them. (You can also check out the breakfast recipes on page 197 for more ideas). Remember: your meal, your choice, as long as it's 1:1:1.

❶❶❶

Slim It Down

Spices are a great way to add interest and even a little sweetness to a meal without adding calories or sugar. Cinnamon in particular has been shown to help stabilize blood sugar levels.

A note about breakfast beverages: one cup of coffee or tea is fine to add to your breakfast. You can even add a little milk and/or sugar if that's how you like your breakfast beverage, but after one cup, switch to water or herbal tea. Too much caffeine can make you hungrier later, and it can also be dehydrating. Drinking caffeinated beverages all day is a good habit to break!

1. Egg sandwich

Protein: 1 scrambled egg prepared with cooking spray in a nonstick skillet.

Carb: 1 English muffin (whole wheat or white).

Fat: 1 ounce cheese.
Alternative: Skip the cheese and spread 1 tablespoon of butter on the English muffin. You can also skip the cheese and spread the English muffin with 1 tablespoon peanut butter and have the egg on the side.

Free foods: Add spinach and chopped tomatoes to the eggs. Or add sliced French breakfast radishes to the egg sandwich for extra crunch.

2. Cottage cheese and berries

Protein: 1 cup cottage cheese. I prefer low-fat varieties.

Carb: 1 cup blueberries (or any other fruit you prefer), mixed into the cottage cheese or served on the side.

Fat: 1 tablespoon chopped walnuts or any other nut. Or try 1 tablespoon of chocolate chips if it's *that* kind of morning.

Free foods: Stir in some cinnamon, nutmeg, cardamom, or any other spice you love to give this breakfast a more interesting or exotic flare.

(continued on page 102)

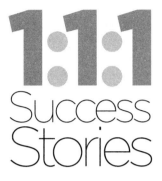

Success Stories

Name: **Yasmine Farazian**
Starting weight: **205 pounds**
Current weight: **145 pounds**
Height: **5'4"**

Weight is as heavy mentally and emotionally as it is physically! If there were a book titled *101 Nicknames for Fat People*, I'd probably recognize every single one of them because I had been fat since I was 5 years old. Some of the names people called me were meant to be terms of endearment (I think?). Others were outright mean. But, hey, as the old saying goes, "Sticks and stones may break my bones, but words will never hurt me," right?

Wrong! Every time someone called me Miss Piggy, Chubs, or Hippo, it was a sting to my psyche. I remember one incident when I was only 10 or 11 and told someone I wanted to take ballet lessons. She scoffed, "They don't have ballet for bears." Then there were the sympathetic glances from strangers, lectures on weight loss from the über-judgmental peanut gallery, and questions from family and friends like: "Why are you doing this? Are you at war with yourself?"

The answer was yes, I was at war with myself, but not because I was overweight. It was because I was unhappy and my pick-me-up of choice was food. Most days, I couldn't wait to get my hands on a doughy and dense loaf of bread, or a crunchy (large) bag of chips and a tub of salty and fatty dip. Eating is what I did to try to feel better.

It's not that I didn't try to lose weight. I did the cabbage soup diet, the lettuce diet, the apple diet, and the Atkins Diet. Jenny Craig and Weight Watchers were just notches on my yo-yo-ing belt! I'd lose 35 pounds, gain 50, lose another 40, and put 60 back on! Exhausted and fed up, I decided to let go, and embrace the fact that I was fat. Defending my overweight status became my pièce de résistance! I was lying to myself in a big way.

Twenty-eight years of food abuse later, I decided to snap out of it. I have tried over and over again to recall my impetus to change. All I remember is sitting at my office desk on a beautiful spring day, clicking open my browser, and typing in "YELP" and searching for "nutritionist." Rania Batayneh's page popped up almost instantly. I clicked on her website link, and the next thing I knew, we had set up our first phone session.

At that session, I was defensive as ever. I told her: "I'm unhappy, I want to lose weight, but I hate dieting, I hate counting calories!"

Rania's response: "Great." She told me I wouldn't have to count a single calorie and she wouldn't dictate what I should eat. Instead, she was going to offer solutions. She explained how her 1:1:1 strategy—one protein, one carb, and one fat at every meal or snack—could change my relationship with food. It was that simple!

I started losing weight right away simply by following the 1:1:1 plan—I lost 13 pounds in the first month! Slowly but surely, I started moving toward changing the habits that weren't in my best inter-est. I began incorporating activities such as long walks with friends, hikes in the hills nearby, and resistance training at the TRX training center, and before long, exercise became second nature. Soon enough, I was so hooked on being active that my body would actually ache if I was inactive for more than 2 days in a row. Within 6 months, I was down 30 pounds.

The change I saw in myself went beyond my new and improved physique. I had a renewed passion for my own life, and my mental and emotional well-being improved. I learned how to say no: no to the unhealthy food choices; no to the people and circumstances that made me uncomfortable; no to anything that made me unhappy! And I also learned how to say yes: to new experiences, to delicious healthy food, and to anything that supported my ultimate goal of being healthy and happy. It took a year, but I dropped 60 pounds and four dress sizes—and I've been at this healthy weight for another year. I'm happier than I've ever been. 1:1:1 not only changed the way I ate, it changed my life.

3. Breakfast burrito

Protein: 1 egg whipped with a little water and cooked like an omelet with cooking spray in a nonstick pan.

Carb: 1 whole grain tortilla. Warm it in a dry skillet, then put it on a plate. Put the egg whites on top.

Fat: 1 ounce feta cheese (you could also use Monterey jack, cheddar, mozzarella or goat cheese). Sprinkle the cheese over the warm egg whites and tortilla and roll it up, burrito style.

Free foods: You can add all kinds of free veggies to a breakfast burrito—sautéed spinach, cherry tomatoes, and/or sliced, lightly sautéed onions and bell peppers are just a few suggestions. A splash of red or green salsa is free, too!

4. Waffles with sausage

Protein: 3 ounces chicken apple sausage.

Carb: 1 waffle with a little syrup. People put syrup on waffles, so I count it as part of the waffle. We're not going to extremes here—you can have a little (1 teaspoon) of syrup if you want it! Or skip it if you don't care about it that much. And by the way, whole grain waffles have more fiber.

Fat: If you use syrup, sprinkle chopped almonds over the waffle for your fat. Or you can use 1 tablespoon of nut butter in place of the syrup. That would be your fat (and it's healthier than the syrup).

Free foods: Top the waffle with some cinnamon. Or chop up your chicken sausages and sauté them with some onions and peppers.

5. Nutty Cereal

Protein: 1 cup low-fat or fat-free milk. If you don't need this much for your cereal, skip it or mix it with coffee to make a latte or with tea and cinnamon to make chai.

Carb: 1 cup cold or hot cereal or $1/_3$ cup granola. It's best to choose one that's high in fiber, at least 5 grams per cup, but if the one you prefer isn't fiber rich, that's okay.

Food for **Thought**

Variety is great, but that doesn't mean you can't eat the same thing every day. If you love a particular breakfast or lunch, then simplify your life and have it every day, or at least every weekday, as long as you still want it and aren't tired of it. If you always want an egg on toast with cheese for breakfast or you love a salad with chicken, almonds, and dried cranberries for lunch, don't force yourself to mix it up. These are fine choices.

Or you can try mixing $1/2$ cup of your favorite sweet cereal with $1/2$ cup of a cereal that's higher in fiber. I'd also encourage you to pick a cereal with no more than 8 grams of sugar per cup—the less the better—but as long as you stick with 1:1:1, I'm not going to insist.

Fat: 1 tablespoon walnuts or other chopped nuts, or 1 tablespoon ground flaxseed.

Free foods: People often want to add fruit to cereal, but that's overdoing the carbs. Move your fruit down to snack time instead (but still have it—it's great for your health!).

6. Protein-boosted oatmeal

Protein: 1 scoop vanilla, chocolate, or unflavored protein powder.

Carb: 1 cup plain cooked oatmeal. Mix the protein powder into your oatmeal.

Fat: 1 tablespoon sliced almonds.

Free foods: Cinnamon or other spices you like.

7. Nutty yogurt

Protein: 6 ounces plain low-fat or nonfat Greek yogurt. Greek yogurt has much more protein than regular yogurt because it's more concentrated.

Carb: 1 teaspoon honey, maple syrup, or agave nectar. If you like your yogurt sweet, it's far better to sweeten it yourself than to buy fruit or flavored yogurt (regular or Greek). They are loaded with sugar. Or skip the sweetener and serve with 1 cup of any chopped fruit (it can be one type or a blend of fruits, as long as you stick to 1 cup), either mixed into the yogurt or on the side.

Fat: 1 tablespoon nut butter or 1 tablespoon chopped nuts. Mixing nut butter into Greek yogurt makes it thicker, almost like a cheesecake—try it!

Free foods: Have some sweet vanilla tea with this breakfast.

Bonus Breakfast: Savory yogurt

Protein: 6 to 8 ounces lowfat or nonfat Greek yogurt.

Carb: Crackers or pita chips on the side or for dipping.

Fat: Mix in 1 tablespoon tahini.

Free foods: Mix chopped cucumbers and scallions with 2 teaspoons lemon juice, and add to the yogurt. Season with sea salt.

Seven 1:1:1 Lunches

Lunch might just be one of the most skipped meals of the day, especially by busy people, but don't skip lunch! This meal keeps you powered up during the time of day when you're expending the most energy. You can have anything you want for lunch—soup, salad, a sandwich, pizza, or something more dinnerlike, if you have the time. Who says you can't have pasta or curry or stir-fry for lunch? Eating heavier foods for lunch and lighter foods for dinner will actually accelerate weight loss because you need more calories during the day when you're moving around, and fewer calories at night translate to more fat burning while you sleep. However, if you like your lunch salad, that's fine, too. Whatever you eat, balance it according to 1:1:1, enjoy an afternoon snack, and you'll make it to the end of the workday without a problem.

1. Mexicali sweet potato

Protein: 1 cup black beans.

Carb: 1 medium sweet potato. Bake it, split it open, and top with the beans.

Fat: $\frac{1}{4}$ of an avocado, cut into slices or cubes.

Free foods: Add salsa, pico de gallo, grilled or sautéed onions, or pickled jalapeño peppers.

2. Turkey sandwich

Protein: 4 to 6 ounces deli turkey.

Carb: 2 slices bread or a 6-inch baguette. Choose whole grain bread most of the time, if you like it.

Fat: $\frac{1}{4}$ of an avocado, 1 tablespoon mayo, or 1 ounce cheese—your choice.

Free foods: Crunch away on all the raw veggies you want. You can also make your sandwich more interesting by adding lettuce, sliced tomato, red onions, pickles, even a splash of hot sauce.

3. Chicken Tortilla Soup (page 237)

Protein: Your protein comes from the chicken in the soup.

Carb: The corn tortillas in the recipe count as the carb. (Or just make regular chicken vegetable soup and top with 1 ounce of crumbled tortilla chips.)

Fat: The recipe includes either avocado or cheece as a topping for the soup—this counts as your fat.

Free foods: Enhance the soup by simmering it with extra veggies, like chopped zucchini, carrots, mushrooms, and/or squash.

4. Salmon Cakes on Mixed Greens (page 238)

Protein: Salmon

Carb: The breadcrumbs in this recipe are the carb.

Fat: 1 ounce crumbled goat cheese over the salad greens. The dressing doesn't count as a fat—I consider dressing part of the salad.

Free foods: Increase the serving size of the mixed greens and/or add other veggies, like chopped broccoli, celery, red bell peppers, and cucumbers.

5. Lunch burrito

Protein: 4 to 6 ounces steak, chicken, or 1 cup black beans.

Carb: 1 flour or 2 small corn tortillas.

Fat: 1 ounce guacamole, cheese, or 1 tablespoon sour cream as a topping or filling—whichever you want the most.

Free foods: Add grilled veggies alongside or inside the burrito.

6. Teriyaki Sesame Chicken (page 229)

Protein: Chicken in the recipe.

Carb: 1 cup cooked white or brown rice, to serve with the chicken.

Fat: Summer Slaw (page 247). Try my recipe, or make this however you want—just combine chopped cabbage with your favorite oily or creamy dressing.

Free foods: Add grated veggies such as carrots and red bell pepper to your rice for more flavor. You could also try shredded broccoli as an alternative or in addition to the shredded cabbage in your coleslaw.

7. Tuna salad on crackers

Protein: 6-ounce can of tuna.

Carb: 1 ounce whole grain crackers

Fat: 1 tablespoon mayo, to mix with the tuna.

Free foods: Add any combination of chopped celery, red onions, bell peppers, pickle relish, and mustard to the tuna.

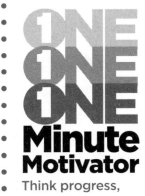

ONE ONE ONE Minute Motivator

Think progress, not perfection!

Seven 1:1:1 Dinners

Some people look forward to dinner all day long because it's the one chance they get to slow down, sit, and really enjoy their food. Dinner should be relaxing. And it doesn't *have* to be all about the food. Enjoy what you're eating, but focus on the other important aspects of the evening meal: winding down at the end of a long day with family or friends, or just having a nice, quiet time by yourself to enjoy the last meal of the day. Dinner is not a time to gorge yourself. Keep it light and simple with 1:1:1!

1. Chicken, baked potato, and grilled veggies

Protein: 6 ounces oven-roasted chicken breast or thighs.

Carb: 1 medium baked potato.

Fat: 1 tablespoon butter or sour cream for the potato.

Free foods: Roasted, grilled, or sautéed vegetables of your choosing. You can also have a big salad if you like.

2. Steak salad

Protein: 4 to 6 ounces filet mignon.

Carb: 1 glass wine (4 ounces). I suggest you save this for after dinner, so it feels extra special.

Fat: 1 tablespoon chopped walnuts or 1 tablespoon bacon bits.

Free foods: Wedge salad (wedge of iceberg lettuce) with 1 tablespoon blue cheese dressing, radishes, and cucumbers. If you like you can serve this with grilled asparagus, steamed mixed squash, or grilled Portobello mushroom slices.

3. Chicken and pasta

Protein: 6 ounces sautéed chicken.

Carb: 1 cup cooked pasta—toss in the chicken if you like them together.

Fat: 1 ounce feta or Pamesan cheese, to sprinkle over the pasta.

Free foods: Add diced canned tomatoes or cherry tomatoes, broccoli florets, artichoke hearts or hearts of palm, and spinach. Add a dash of cayenne pepper for a kick.

4. Raspberry spinach salad with salmon

Protein: 6-ounce salmon filet (or any other baked or grilled fish).

Carb: 1 cup lentiis.

Fat: 1 tablespoon pistachios.

Free foods: 2 cups baby spinach (with raspberry vinaigrette). Add jicama and radishes to your salad, for flavor and crunch.

5. Greek Pasta Salad with White Beans
(page 209)

Protein: White beans.

Carb: Pasta.

Fat: Feta cheese.

Free foods: Add eggplant, zucchini, and/or squash to the salad.

6. Butternut Squash Curry (page 216)

Protein: The chicken or the chickpeas in the recipe count as your protein.

Carb: 1 cup couscous.

Fat: Almonds

Free foods: Try adding more veggies to this curry, like cauliflower florets, more bell peppers (try green, yellow, orange, and red), and chopped bok choy or kale.

7. Thai Chicken Noodle Dinner (page 223)

Protein: Chicken

Carb: Rice noodles.

Fat: Peanut butter used to make the sauce.

Free foods: Add more veggies to this recipe to make it more filling. Try cilantro, shredded carrots, and a little bit of cayenne pepper for spice. You could also add chopped scallions to your garnish.

Seven 1:1:1 Snacks

Snacks are crucial for success on the 1:1:1 plan, so you never get overly hungry and you can stick to your balanced plan at meals. Don't skip your midmorning and midafternoon snacks!

Snack #1

Protein: 1 string cheese.

Carb: $\frac{1}{2}$ ounce baked chips.

Fat: 1 tablespoon sour cream dip with fresh chopped herbs.

Free foods: Raw broccoli florets.

Snack #2

Protein: 2 to 3 ounces deli turkey.

Carb: 1 apple.

Fat: 1 tablespoon peanut butter, to spread on the apple.

Free foods: Sliced radishes or jicama sticks.

Snack #3

Protein: $\frac{1}{2}$ cup hummus.

Carb: $\frac{1}{2}$ pita, cut into wedges for dipping.

Fat: $\frac{1}{4}$ of an avocado.

Free foods: Raw cauliflower florets.

Snack #4

Protein: 1 hard-cooked egg.
Carb: ½ ounce whole grain crackers.
Fat: 1-ounce cheese wedge to spread on the crackers.
Free foods: Celery sticks.

Snack #5

Protein: 6 ounces Greek yogurt.
Carb: 2 tablespoons granola.
Fat: 1 tablespoon dark chocolate chips.
Free foods: Green or peppermint tea.

Snack #6

Protein: 3 ounces roasted chicken.
Carb: ½ bagel.
Fat: ½ cup hummus.
Free foods: Baby carrots.

Snack #7

Protein: 1 ounce feta cheese.
Carb: ½ ounce pita chips.
Fat: 10 small olives.
Free foods: Chopped tomatoes (mix with feta and olives as a dip for the pita chips).

———————

I hope you're fully inspired now, and feeling more comfortable constructing your meals and snacks according to 1:1:1. Your only limit is your own creativity. Try new foods as often as you can. But most importantly, relax and enjoy every bite. You know you're eating right, so you don't have to worry!

CHAPTER SEVEN

1:1:1
Accelerated

The 1:1:1 plan will keep anyone in balance, and if you're an overeater or an unbalanced eater, or if you have quite a lot of weight to lose, 1:1:1 is all you need. At least for now. However.

Some people want to go a little further, push themselves a little more, and are motivated to lose weight a little faster. Maybe they want a jump start, or, they've been dieting for a while and they've hit a plateau. They need to break through. Or they love rules, crave rules, and want *more rules*. Maybe they only have a few pounds left to lose and those last few aren't coming off so easily.

If you can relate to any of these scenarios, then 1:1:1 Accelerated is for you.

1:1:1 Accelerated is still 1:1:1, but with the belt tightened just a little. It has a few more strategies, a few additional things to keep in mind, and some tricks up its sleeve. Fortunately, the changes are small and the payoff is big. People who do 1:1:1 Accelerated can expect to see speedier, more dramatic weight loss, and who doesn't want that? It's great for chronic dieters who are already eating a fairly low-calorie diet and need to try something new, as well as for people who have fewer than 20 pounds to lose. (Weight loss gets harder the closer you are to your goal!)

In this chapter, I'll explain in detail each of these new 1:1:1 Accelerated strategies, but here's a preview—seven slimming strategies to accelerate your weight loss.

1. You won't eat starchy carbs after your afternoon snack. This is a big adjustment for some people, but when you get used to it, it becomes a way of life. Normally vegetables are "free," but on 1:1:1 Accelerated, vegetables become your official carb at dinner—your only carb. However, you may have as large a serving of vegetables as you like. You can still have starches like bread and pasta and sweets like fruit and cookies, but on the Accelerated plan, you must have these earlier in the day only.

2. You'll make double-doers do double duty: If a food is a carb and a protein (like beans), a protein and a fat (like cheese), or a carb and a fat (like chocolate), you'll count that food as both categories in the same meal.

3. You'll never have any food more than once a day, except for vegetables. This is particularly important with a few specific foods: cheese, bread, nuts, nut butter, chocolate, coffee, and meal replacement bars or shakes. Once you've had one portion, that's it for the day. You need to choose something different for your next meal or snack.

4. One slice of bread is a portion, even with a sandwich—go topless!

5. Those easygoing exceptions for 1:1:1 are no longer. You're tightening the reins! From now on, salad dressing doesn't just come with the salad—it counts as a fat serving. Syrup doesn't just come with your pancakes—it counts as a carb (so put nut butter on your pancakes instead). Likewise, cream in your coffee is now officially a fat serving.

6. You can have a glass of wine or other alcoholic beverage, a dessert, or a cheat dinner with a starchy carb once a week. When you do this, simply cut your starchy or sweet carb from your lunch—veggie carbs only allow you more leeway for your "cheat" dinner. And you thought this would be hard!

7. You'll officially count baked goods like cookies, muffins, and cake not just as a carb, but as a carb and a fat. (Like you always knew they were!)

Yes, it's tougher. Yes, it's stricter. But if you're having trouble losing weight, you've hit a plateau, you've been a low-carb dieter, or you just can't get rid of those last 5 to 15 pounds, 1:1:1 Accelerated may be what you need to break through to your goal. Use 1:1:1 Accelerated when you need it, and once you reach your weight loss goal, you can go back to regular 1:1:1 if you want to be a bit less strict. (Or you can stay on 1:1:1 Accelerated for as long as you like—there's nothing wrong with it as a lifestyle.)

Which 1:1:1 approach is right for you? The flowchart on pages 112–113 will help you figure it out.

I have many clients who do just fine on the regular 1:1:1 plan, but I also can easily spot the ones who are going to do better on 1:1:1 Accelerated once I look at their first food diary. As soon as I recognize them, I immediately bring up this option.

For example, I have a client named Lucy who did Weight Watchers for months and lost 30 pounds, but then her weight loss stalled. She still wanted to lose at least 18 more pounds and she was staying within her points, so she couldn't figure out why she wasn't losing any more weight. She came to me to find out why.

It was obvious from her food diary. She was eating mostly popcorn, bread, and desserts, and very little protein. Lucy was definitely out of balance. I also noticed a telltale diet killer: Every night, she had a Weight Watchers éclair before bed! I suggested that Lucy try 1:1:1 Accelerated, particularly because it would break her of that evening éclair habit. I suggested that she have that éclair as part of a midafternoon snack once a week on a weekday and then again just once on the

(continued on page 114)

WHICH 1:1:1 APPROACH SHOULD I CHOOSE?

START HERE

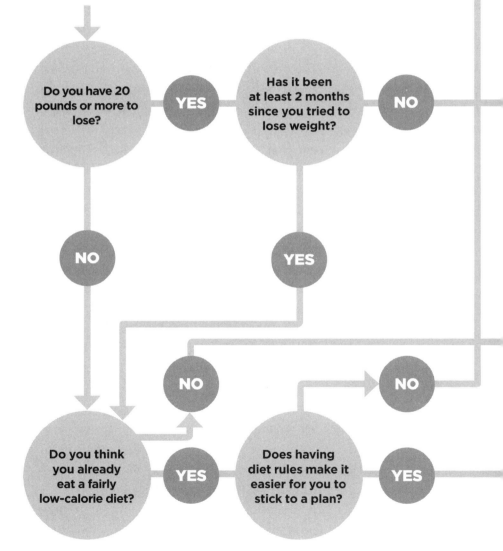

Do you have 20 pounds or more to lose?

YES

Has it been at least 2 months since you tried to lose weight?

NO

NO

YES

NO

NO

Do you think you already eat a fairly low-calorie diet?

YES

Does having diet rules make it easier for you to stick to a plan?

YES

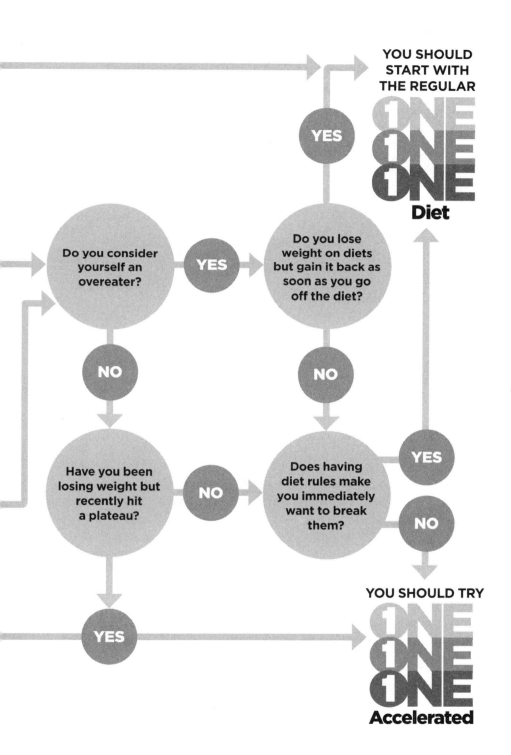

weekend, during the day. At first she thought she'd never be able to adjust. Turns out, she adjusted quite well! She always knew that éclair was coming in a few days, and she wasn't nearly as hungry as she used to be because she was balancing her protein, carbs, and fat, instead of

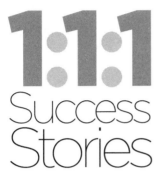

Name: **Byron Jarnagin**
Starting weight : **223 pounds**
Current weight: **198 pounds**
Height: **5'7"**

Name: **Josie Jarnagin**
Starting weight: **152 pounds**
Current weight: **135 pounds**
Height: **5'3"**

Byron says:

I had always gone through healthy spurts where I'd exercise and eat well and lose weight, but then I'd stop and gain it all back. During my unhealthy phases, I ate a lot of junk food, and soda was my stress reliever. About a year ago, it hit me that every shirt, jacket, and pair of pants I bought was size XL. Looking back at pictures from the prior year or two, I could see how heavy I'd become.

Still, I admit seeing a nutritionist was my wife's idea. Even so, sessions with Rania helped me see food differently. It was a big deal to me to not have to restrict my food choices; I just needed to be conscious of pairings and quantity. In just 6 months, my waist size went from 40" to 36", and I dropped 25 pounds. I had to buy new clothes, and it felt great to be in a smaller size. I'm now focused on being more consistent with my exercise routine so I can reach my goal weight of 185 pounds, but I'm going to follow the 1:1:1 approach for life.

focusing on mostly carbs. She also lost those last 18 pounds in just over 2 months.

Then there's Sam. The majority of foods he ate were very low in calories and he was working out with a trainer, but he couldn't get rid of

---

Josie says:

I used to dread Monday mornings. I'd worry about what I was going to wear to work. Would it fit? Would it be comfortable? I wanted to lose weight, but I knew I couldn't do it without the support of my husband. Plus, he needed to slim down, too. None of the diet plans I knew about seemed right for us. They were overwhelming. I wanted something I could do with Byron and our 3-year old, so the whole family would be eating the same way. That's why I decided to consult a nutritionist, and I'm glad we found Rania.

Our sessions with Rania are simple and fast. We discuss our weekly food logs and determine where to tweak things. I love sugar and Rania has helped me keep my sugar, but in smaller quantities. I still eat cookies, ice cream, doughnuts, and hot chocolate, but I've lost more than 17 pounds in 6 months. I did this without counting points, calories, or carbs or spending hours in the gym. (I do walk 20 minutes a day, though.) Rania gave us great snack ideas and recipes. She gets that my husband and I have different taste-buds and has given us ideas to help us work around that so the same meal satisfies both of us. For example, we make chicken fajitas now—I don't like spicy food but my husband does, so we add a little bit of seasoning, set aside a portion for me and for leftovers, then add a lot of seasoning for my husband. We do the same for dishes with sauces—add a little, set aside a portion for me, then add the rest of the sauce for him. One dish and we are both satisfied! Now on Monday mornings, when my clothes don't fit, it's usually because they're too big!

those last 10 pounds. He was building lots of muscle, but his "love handles" persisted. When I switched him to 1:1:1 Accelerated, the fat melted off in 6 weeks and he reached his goal weight. No more love handles!

Yet another client, a low-carb aficionado named Barb, gained weight every time she looked at a piece of toast (or so she said). Her body had adjusted to a low-carb lifestyle, so starchy foods caused immediate bloating and weight gain. But even when she was eating low-carb, she had completely stopped losing and couldn't get rid of the last 17 pounds. (Her goal was to get back to the weight she'd been at her wedding 11 years earlier.) Barb was also terrified to do 1:1:1 because of the carb serving at every meal. I suggested she try 1:1:1 Accelerated, because one of the key rules is that for dinner, starchy carbs are forbidden. Protein, fat, and vegetables only! Barb decided that maybe she could get back into balance if she ate carbs during the day when she was active, but not at night. Sure enough, within 8 weeks, Barb could have fit into her wedding dress!

The changes for 1:1:1 Accelerated are simple but powerful and they'll supercharge your weight loss. However, 1:1:1 Accelerated isn't all work and no play—you get a cheat dinner every week, so you don't ever feel too deprived and you can accommodate special events like dinner parties or restaurant meals. The rules are basically the same when you opt for 1:1:1 Accelerated. You'll still have breakfast, a midmorning snack, lunch, a midafternoon snack, and a satisfying dinner. You'll still balance your meals and snacks according to 1:1:1. But let's look more closely at the seven new strategies you'll layer on top of what you're already doing with 1:1:1.

Accelerated Strategy #1: Make Dinner Different

It's always 1:1:1, right? There's one exception. On 1:1:1 Accelerated, at dinner there's a slight change. All those nonstarchy vegetables that used to be free are no longer free after your afternoon snack. In fact, now they're officially carbs. Another difference: you don't have to limit yourself to one type of nonstarchy vegetable the way you have to choose between pasta, rice, or potatoes on regular 1:1:1. You can still have as many as you want in whatever portion size you want—you can still have steamed broccoli or grilled asparagus or sautéed Brussels sprouts *and* a salad, if you so desire. But bread, pasta, rice, fruit, or dessert? Nope. Off the dinner menu.

This isn't really such a stretch. You probably already know that all vegetables contain some carbohydrates. The amount of carbohydrates in vegetables isn't significant, which is why you can still eat them on the 1:1:1 plan and also have something starchy like bread, pasta, rice, sweet potatoes, or something else with a higher carbohydrate count from sugar, like fruit or dessert. But if you want to lose weight faster, you need to cut back on starchy carbs. That's why eating vegetable carbs only at dinner is the biggest, most important rule for 1:1:1 Accelerated.

So here's how to do this. You might have a nice, juicy steak and a big pile of yummy asparagus topped with lemon butter. Your steak is the protein, your asparagus is the carb, and your lemon butter is the fat. That's dinner, and that's enough. Another example: You could have a big bowl of chili with lots of vegetables, like onions, peppers, and zucchini, as well as ground turkey—but no beans. Top it off with some sour cream (fat) and enjoy! Or how about a nice roasted chicken breast sliced into a big bowl of mixed greens and raw veggies and drizzled with your favorite toasted sesame dressing? Delicious!

The reason getting your dinnertime carbs from vegetables accelerates weight loss is the same reason I recommend never having an evening snack: Your body recovers and repairs during the night while you sleep. Don't overwhelm it with starchy carbs or sugars at night. If you don't provide that fuel, your body will have to find another source to burn. What's left? Your fat stores. With this switch, you're just *accelerating* your fat burn.

At first, some of my clients complain about this. How can they give up carbs at night? What's dinner without pasta or dessert? I totally get the sacrifice, and if you want to have those things, stick with regular 1:1:1. You'll still slim down, but maybe not as quickly, especially if you're just a few pounds from your goal weight. It's up to you whether you want to accelerate your weight loss. However, remember this: If you aren't losing weight the way you would like, something you're doing isn't working well enough. If you want to lose weight, you're going to have to change something. I know from experience that this is a highly effective change to make. Besides, it's not like you can't ever eat bread or pasta or dessert or wine again. You can have all those things. Just not at dinner.

Also, skipping starchy carbs at night isn't as hard as you might think. Balancing all your meals and snacks according to 1:1:1 will reduce your cravings and you won't be starving by dinnertime, or afterwards. Or ever. You will be balanced, so you 'll never feel frantic or deprived.

Accelerated Strategy #2: Make Double-Doers Do Double Duty

Normally, double-doers are foods that can be counted toward one of two categories, depending on what else you want to have in your meal. So for instance, cheese could be your fat in a sandwich with turkey (protein) or it could be your protein in a fresh mozzarella sandwich

Food for **Thought**

Diet soda may seem like the perfect way to round out a 1:1:1 snack, but think again. Research suggests that diet soda actually increases cravings for sweet foods. You may end up eating more later, just because you had that diet soda. One study by the University of Texas revealed that study participants who drank more than two diet sodas per day had a 70 percent greater waist circumference than those who abstained from the fake stuff. Plus diet soda contains ingredients proven to cause several kinds of cancer in mice. No thanks! Instead, choose club soda with a squeeze of lemon, lime, or orange—all the bubbles, none of the creepy chemicals!

with basil olive oil (fat). On 1:1:1 Accelerated, however, double-doers take on a new role: They literally do double duty in the same meal. If you have a double-doer in your meal, that one food will do two jobs. Go back to Chapter 4 and check for the list of foods with superscripts: the protein foods that can also be fats (cheese, whole eggs) or carbs (beans, peas, and legumes); the carb foods that can also be proteins (quinoa and legumes) or fats (ice cream and chocolate); and the fat foods that can also be proteins (hummus) or carbs (French fries or other deep fat fried food). When you choose any of those double-doers on the Accelerated plan, it counts as your serving for two categories.

For example, if you choose a sandwich for lunch, choose the turkey or the cheese, but not both. The cheese can stand in as a protein and a fat because it's a double-doer. (The turkey isn't a double-doer, however, so if you choose the turkey, you can also add mayonnaise or avocado for your fat. You might as well throw on some lettuce and tomato, while you're at it.)

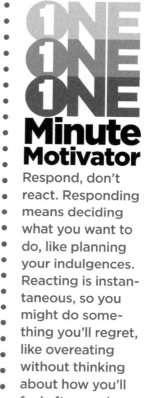

Minute Motivator

Respond, don't react. Responding means deciding what you want to do, like planning your indulgences. Reacting is instantaneous, so you might do something you'll regret, like overeating without thinking about how you'll feel afterward.

Accelerated Strategy #3: Stick with One of Everything

The next strategy is simple: Never have any food more than once per day. On the 1:1:1 plan, you could have toast for breakfast and a sandwich for lunch if that's what you really wanted. However, on 1:1:1 Accelerated, if you have the toast or the sandwich, you need to make a different, bread-free carb choice at your next meal. If you had toast for breakfast, make fruit or beans your carb at lunch. If you want a sandwich for lunch, make fruit your breakfast carb of choice.

This applies to every food item (except vegetables), but most importantly, it applies to a few particular foods. Make sure you only have one portion per day (max) of these foods:

- Bread
- Cheese
- Nuts
- Nut butter
- Chocolate

- Coffee (let cup number two be herbal tea, to moderate your caffeine intake)
- Meal replacement shakes or bars

This strategy forces you to mix up your protein, carb, and fat choices and prevents you from making high-fat or high-calorie foods like cheese or nut butter or high-carb foods like bread your go-to choices. If you can't have them, you automatically add more variety to your diet, and the options are often less caloric, lower in fat, and/or lower in carbs. Even if they aren't, you'll be getting a wider variety of nutrients, which can help you feel more satisfied and more energetic. For example, if you're used to eating cheese at every meal, you'll need to choose some other fat option, like walnuts or olive oil. If you're used to eating bread at every meal, have brown rice or fruit.

The nice thing about this rule is that you can still have any food you want. You can still have chocolate or cheese or almond butter. You just can't go overboard. Technically, on 1:1:1, you could eat cheese or chocolate at every meal (although I hope you won't!). If it helps to write down what you eat so you remember whether you already had bread or cheese or chocolate or nuts, then go for it.

Accelerated Strategy #4: Go Topless or Bottomless!

If you want bread, you have one slice, not two. You can still have a sandwich but make it open-faced. You're trimming.

This is a great rule because, once again, there's no restriction. You can have all those foods you love. You're just cutting back the amount a bit, to reduce the calorie count here and there, where you'll hardly notice.

Accelerated Strategy #5: Tighten the Reins

On the standard 1:1:1 plan, certain things become part of the food. For instance, syrup counts as part of a waffle, flavored oatmeal counts as part of the oatmeal, cream counts as part of the coffee, and salad dressing counts as part of the salad. Those days are over! It's time to tighten up the reins. On 1:1:1 Accelerated, syrup is a separate carb, so choose nut butter with your waffle instead of syrup. Flavored oatmeal is two carbs (oatmeal

Food for **Thought**

Everywhere I go, once people find out I'm a nutritionist, they always ask me the same question: "What's the *one* thing I can do to start losing weight?" I love this question because it's such an easy way to introduce the concept of "one."

I usually ask, "What's the one thing you know you shouldn't be doing?" When they tell me, I tell them a way to cut it down to one. For example, if they eat sweets too often, I tell them to cut down to *one* sweet per day. If they do something every day, like eat fried food, I tell them to cut down to *one* serving of french fries per week. Whatever *they* believe is their dietary Achilles heel, that's where I focus my *one* therapy!

An airport driver once answered my question by saying, "I eat cheese too much."

"How much?" I asked.

"At every meal," he admitted.

My answer: "The *one* thing you can do is to eat cheese at just *one* meal per day."

Four months later, I got him as a driver again because I always use the same service when I fly to and from Los Angeles. He was excited to see me because he wanted to tell me that my advice had started him on a great path, and he had lost 25 pounds. That's the power of *one!*

and sugar), so get the plain stuff and add cinnamon instead for a hint of sweetness. As for your salad, the dressing counts, so either skip it, use a fat-free substitute like salsa, or forego the other fatty adds like cheese, nuts, or avocados in favor of a good dressing. Just choose the one fat you want.

Once again, there is no restriction, just a slight narrowing of choices at any given meal. You can always have the thing you pass on next time, so don't worry about feeling like you can never have something you love again. (Plus, once you've reached your goal, you can go back to regular 1:1:1 for maintenance—and your little flavored packets of oatmeal will be back on the menu!)

Accelerated Strategy #6: Limit Your Treats to Once a Week

When you're trying hard to lose weight, a few things can really foil your progress, like alcohol, desserts, even those beloved carbs at dinner. Instead of banning those entirely on 1:1:1 Accelerated, all you have to do is limit them to once a week.

If you have an event or a date or happening where you know you'll want to have a glass of wine or a cocktail, that's fine. Reserve that day as your one cheat day, and enjoy a glass. (Of course, you don't ever have to have an alcoholic drink at all. This is only if you really want one.)

Sometimes, you just can't pass up that chocolate mousse, or you go to a restaurant with a to-die-for creme brulee, or your date insists on splitting the strawberry sundae. You can join in! Just keep it to once a week. Pick the day you'll get the most pleasure out of your dessert, and savor it. You can do it again next week! (As with alcohol, you can also choose not to have a weekly dessert. I'm not going to force tiramisu down your throat! Or be super virtuous and skip all that stuff! Up to you.) Or, maybe you're in someone's home and she's serving her signature lasagna for dinner, or everyone decides to order pizza and you don't want to be the one person who spoils the party by saying, "Um, I can't actually eat that." No problem! So—one cheat a week. Alcohol, dessert, or starchy carb. Got it? However, if you go a week or two without a cheat meal? Even better. Cheating is definitely not required, but it is allowed. Once. However, on your cheat day, give yourself some wiggle room. Make lunch your meal with veggie-only carbs. Easy!

Accelerated Strategy #7: Turn Baked Goods into Double-Doers

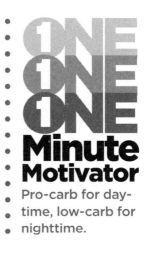

ONE ONE ONE Minute Motivator

Pro-carb for daytime, low-carb for nighttime.

On the 1:1:1 plan, sweet, sugary baked goods like cookies, muffins, chocolate croissants, and cake count as a carb, period. However, we all know that baked goods contain a lot of fat, so on 1:1:1 Accelerated, these are officially double-doers: carb and fat. You can have a muffin for breakfast, but skip the butter. Have a cookie, but don't worry about pairing it with a fat. You don't have to deprive yourself of your favorite bakery treats—just acknowledge their fat content, enjoy them, and move on.

That's it! Follow these seven Accelerated slimming strategies, and the weight will start peeling off. The regular 1:1:1 balance still applies—every meal and every snack includes one serving each of protein, carbs, and fat. Just add these eight simple strategies, and you'll see success.

A lot of my clients really enjoy the 1:1:1 Accelerated plan, once they get into the habit. It works fast, it feels good, it's clear and easy to follow, and you can sustain it in the real world without feeling like you have to miss out on anything. You still get to eat the foods you want. You just eat them within this particular structure.

1:1:1 Accelerated Food Diary

Back in Chapter 5, I decoded some of my clients' food diaries for you. In this chapter, I want to show you how I would comment on a food diary for someone on 1:1:1 Accelerated. Meet Michele! Michele is a 34-year-old female who has successfully lost 29 pounds on 1:1:1 and had 11 more to lose. She stayed consistent with her workouts but found that her weight wasn't changing, so we discussed how she could incorporate 1:1:1

Michelle's Accelerated Diary

	Breakfast	Snack
Monday	1 English muffin with 1 ounce cheese *Good job counting the cheese as your "double-doer," acting as both a protein and a fat for this meal. Another option: Top your English muffin with 1 egg.*	1 cup blueberries + $^3/_4$ cup plain Greek yogurt + 1 tablespoon almonds *This is a perfect Accelerated snack.*

Accelerated into her weight loss journey. She lost the last 11 pounds in 5 weeks. That's how fast it works! Here are 3 days out of her food diary, with my notes:

Lunch	Snack	Dinner
Chicken sandwich on 1 slice bread with avocado slices and tons of veggies	1 banana + 1 cup milk + 1 tablespoon dark chocolate chips	At sushi restaurant: 6 pieces sashimi + cucumber salad
You did this right! One of the rules of the Accelerated plan is to only have one of each food in your day. This adds variety. Making the simple swap from cheese to avocado fits this rule, since you had cheese for breakfast. (And avocados are great for your heart and memory!) Also, good job scaling back your bread to one slice.	*This is a great Accelerated snack that adds something sweet to the mix so you don't feel deprived.*	*This is an excellent Accelerated dinner. The sashimi gives you plenty of protein and the cucumber salad with dressing is your carb and fat. Good choice passing on sushi rolls, which contain rice and are therefore not appropriate for dinner on 1:1:1 Accelerated (unless of course it's your one weekly cheat night).*

(continued)

Michelle's Accelerated Diary—Continued

	Breakfast	**Snack**
Tuesday	Oatmeal + 1 scoop vanilla protein powder + 1 tablespoon walnuts + cinnamon *This is a great tweak to your usual flavored oatmeal. The oatmeal is your carb, protein powder is your protein, and walnuts are your fat. The cinnamon and the protein powder add flavor without sugar.*	1 sliced apple + 1 tablespoon almond butter + 1/2 ounce turkey jerky *This well-rounded snack will keep you going until lunch*
Wednesday	1 frozen waffle + 1 tablespoon almond butter + 1 slice turkey bacon *Good job using almond butter instead of the syrup, which would be an extra carb on 1:1:1 Accelerated.*	1 cup cottage cheese mixed with banana slices, cinnamon, and 1 tablespoon almonds *This is a good snack!*

Lunch	Snack	Dinner
1 slice cheese pizza + mixed green salad with ranch dressing	5 whole grain cracker crisps with ½ cup hummus + tomatoes and cucumber	Grilled lamb chops with roasted veggies
Pizza makes perfect. This is an all-in-one protein, carb, and fat because the cheese is a double-doer. Another rule on the Accelerated plan is to pare it down to one, however, so with the cheese and the dressing, you've got a double fat (even though the cheese is also a protein). Instead of ranch dressing, drizzle balsamic vinegar over your salad, but enjoy tons of salad veggies to fill you up.	*I like how you added filling veggies.*	*This is another great Accelerated meal. The roasted veggies are your carb. Keep up the good work!*
1 cup chicken tortilla soup with a dollop sour cream	Hard-cooked egg + 1 mini whole wheat pita	Black bean burger, no bun, with avocado + grilled veggies on the side
The soup is your protein (chicken) and carb (tortilla). The fat is the sour cream. Well done. Skipping the cheese and going for sour cream is a good strategy, but next time, you could choose the cheese instead, just to switch things up.	*Good job—the egg is your protein/fat combo. Fill up on raw veggies for crunch and fiber if this isn't enough for you.*	*Skipping the bun at night is the perfect way to accelerate your weight loss. Black beans are a great source of protein and avocado is your fat. Grilled veggies serve as your carb and they're a great way to add variety (and fiber!) to any meal.*

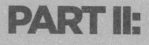

PART II

1:1:1 in the REAL WORLD

CHAPTER EIGHT
Living 1:1:1

You'd be hard-pressed to find an approach to healthy eating that's easier than 1:1:1. Still, I'm sure you have questions. Many clients ask me how to handle particular scenarios, wonder about certain kinds of foods, and aren't sure how to manage particular real-life situations. In this chapter, you'll find answers to some of the most common questions about applying the 1:1:1 plan, so you can live the lifestyle like you mean it and lose the weight you don't want to carry around with you anymore.

Q If I can choose any food I want for 1:1:1, I'm afraid I won't choose healthy foods. What if I end up just eating cheeseburgers, pizza, and cookies with milk? Won't I develop a nutritional deficiency?

A One of the main reasons why people go off diets is that they feel deprived, so the great thing about 1:1:1 is that you are never forbidden from eating any of your favorite foods. If you're dying for some chocolate, you can choose it as your carb. If you have to have a cheeseburger, then enjoy it because the bun (carb), burger (protein), and cheese (fat) fit into 1:1:1. Don't worry so much about always picking the "best" option. Pick the one you really want. If the "healthiest" choice sounds good to you, have it, but if it doesn't, then have something you want more. Otherwise, you'll feel deprived and overeat. The freedom that comes with 1:1:1 is your key to staying balanced and not falling off the wagon.

Many of my clients who are chronic overeaters need the simple restraint that 1:1:1 provides, before they can think about anything else. This gets weight loss started in a big way. If you're used to eating fries, soda, and cookies with your cheeseburger, than choosing just the cheeseburger will cut your calorie intake by quite a lot, and it will help get your system back into balance.

That's when the magic happens. I see it time and time again. The better you start to feel, and the faster the weight comes off, the more you'll find yourself choosing healthier options. You'll start to crave healthier food, as your body gets to a healthier state. One day, you may realize that you'd rather have the veggie pizza than the cheeseburger. Maybe a crisp, juicy apple suddenly sounds better than a cookie. Knowing you can *always choose the cookie* when you want to may be enough to free you up to choose the apple on occasion—and then you'll start to feel even better, and at some point, you may recognize that you actually like feeling better, and soon cookies will be a distant memory. You want to keep feeling good, and that good feeling eventually overpowers the momentary pleasure of a candy bar on the tongue. You might even start to crave vegetables!

An important part of the 1:1:1 plan is trust. You're trusting your own body to balance and heal as you begin to feed it in a healthier way. It's an exciting, free-spirited way to "diet," which is exactly why it works. You can always have the cheeseburger, the pizza, the cookie. You can always skip the salad. But aim for making the

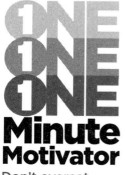

ONE ONE ONE Minute Motivator

Don't overeat, then dash off to the gym to burn off the calories and guilt. Eat just what your body needs, so "burning it off" happens naturally. No gym required.

healthy choice most of the time, and you may find yourself ordering that salad after all.

Q A lot of diets tell you to give up coffee. I would never give up coffee. Can I have coffee on the 1:1:1 plan?

A Of course. You can have anything you want on the 1:1:1 plan, as long as it's in balance, and I would never take your beloved cup of coffee away from you if you really want it. However, while coffee isn't going to kill you or make you fat, it's not a great idea to drink too much of it. While coffee has antioxidants, the additives like cream and sugar and flavored syrup and whipped cream can add too many calories and too much sugar and fat to your diet, and even the effects of too much black coffee may be harmful. A Duke University study demonstrated that coffee consumption can actually hinder the body's ability to regulate insulin and glucose levels in the blood in those with type-2 diabetes. Insulin and blood sugar are closely related to your appetite, and drinking anything that messes with that system isn't a good idea, as far as I'm concerned.

Tea is full of healthful antioxidants, so why not swap your second cup of coffee for a cup of black or green tea? Tea has caffeine, too, but not as much, so it may help you "step down" a caffeine addiction. If you need more comforting beverages, then switch to herbal tea or an unsweetened plain or flavored iced tea. There are so many yummy flavors of herbal tea that hydrate you without jolting your body with caffeine. These teas can even stand in for dessert. Try apple cinnamon, orange spice, peppermint, chamomile, or even vanilla or chocolate tea instead of a nighttime snack.

In the meantime, if a cup of joe gets you going in the morning, then go for it. You can even add cream and a teaspoon of sugar, since you're just having the one cup (on 1:1:1, I consider these parts of the coffee). For that matter, you can even have your fancy mocha latte or caramel macchiato —just recognize that if you have one of these large, fancy coffee drinks, you may have a complete 1:1:1 snack covered: milk is a protein, whipped cream is a fat, and sugar is a carb. (So skip the giant muffin!)

Q So, 1:1:1. I get it. Everything in my meal should be 1:1:1. So I can have spaghetti (carb) with meatballs (protein) and Parmesan cheese (fat), plus garlic bread (carb) with butter (fat) and cheese (protein), plus a salad with croutons (carb), bacon bits (protein), and shredded cheese (fat), right?

A Nice try. If you have the cheese bread for breakfast, the spaghetti for lunch, and the salad for dinner, you're good to go, but each meal is 1:1:1, not each individual element of the meal. If you have steak (protein), asparagus with Hollandaise sauce (fat), and a sweet potato (carb), plus a salad with croutons (carb), cheese (fat), and bacon bits (protein), you've gone over. Don't double up on any meal or snack. Don't have the lobster and the shrimp, the bread and the wine, or the cheese and the avocado. It's either/or. One means one.

Q Can I be a vegetarian and still follow 1:1:1?

A Of course! Vegetarian, vegan, pescatarian, flexitarian—whatever you call yourself, 1:1:1 still works perfectly well. Let's say you want veggie pizza. The crust is your carb, the cheese is your protein, and add olives to your pizza for fat or have a side salad with avocado or olives. In a veggie sandwich with cheese, the bread is the carb, the cheese is the protein, and you might choose hummus for your fat. If you're a vegan, you might find yourself trying to figure out how to manage tofu, veggie burgers, tempeh, and other plant proteins. Those are just what they say: proteins! Choose one, add a carb like a whole grain, a fat like olive oil, avocado, or nuts, and plenty of free veggies. Easy!

Q I love to eat. Am I going to get to eat enough food on 1:1:1?

A If you're an overeater, or in particular a carb overeater, you're probably accustomed to eating more food than you need. Simple carbs like sugar and white flour are among the world's most powerful appetite stimulants! When you're in balance, you won't be able to eat a whole bag of chips or a whole box of cookies. That would make you feel sick. But if you're used to eating tons of carbs, that's what can happen. You learn to eat more and more and more because you're always hungry. Similarly, If you're used to stuffing yourself until you're uncomfortably full, you may need to readjust to eating an appropriate amount, but that's in your best interest. If you're an over-eater, you've been eating too much food, and it's better for your waist-line as well as your digestion to get back into the habit of eating just what your body requires to function. The 1:1:1 plan is the perfect way to do this without being deprived. You should feel satisfied but not stuffed after a good meal. Many of my clients report that at first, they feel like they aren't eating enough because they aren't stuffed. But once they get used to how much better they feel after a smaller meal, they report preferring the 1:1:1-sized meal to what they used to eat. You'll be surprised when you start following 1:1:1 how filling a smaller meal with the right combination of protein, fat, and carbs will be.

Also remember that on 1:1:1, you eat three meals and two snacks. This is why you're able to eat less at each meal and still feel satisfied—you're eating frequently! Think about your lunch yesterday. Were you so full that you skipped your afternoon snack and then felt famished on your drive home so you turned into the fast-food place and went through the drive-thru? After lunch, remind yourself that you'll be getting a snack in just a few hours. Can you wait a few hours? I bet you can.

Finally, never forget that vegetables are free. If you're truly hungry, make your meal more filling with a salad, or any raw or cooked nonstarchy vegetables: broccoli, cauliflower, celery, carrots, cabbage, Brussels sprouts, asparagus, green or red bell peppers, or a nice sliced tomato. Eat to your heart's content.

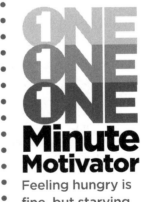

ONE ONE ONE Minute Motivator

Feeling hungry is fine, but starving is not. Never let yourself get to the point of feeling famished, or you'll be much more likely to overeat.

Q Can I have a nighttime snack?

A I use an acronym for after-dinner snacks: ADS. I call them ADS because they can *add* a lot of calories and fat to your day. Your body needs time to settle down and digest your dinner, then ease into sleep mode. It doesn't need to be digesting popcorn and cookies and crackers and cheese right before bedtime. You don't need all those calories when you sleep. You need them during the day when you're running around. Calories your body doesn't need get turned into fat you don't want.

If you're in the habit of eating at night, it might be just that: a habit. If you get used to doing something different during that time, like checking social media or doing a word or number puzzle, or even doing situps while you watch reality TV, then you might not miss that nighttime snack at all.

You might also be hungry at night because you didn't eat enough during the day. Did you skip any of your other snacks? Have them earlier, not at night. Did you eat full portion sizes of all three components of 1:1:1 for every meal? This is key to feeling satisfied.

However, some people enjoy eating or drinking a little something after dinner, to complete the meal. If that's you, then just save part of your dinner for later. You could save your carb option from dinner and make it your dessert. A piece of fruit is your best bet, but even a glass of wine or an ounce of dark chocolate is okay, as long as it was your dinner carb, not an add-on carb. If you can get by without it, however, skipping the nighttime snack is the ideal way to encourage your body to burn fat while you sleep.

Q Can I split my portions into half portions so I can have more things? Like, can I have half a portion of blueberries and half a portion of granola in my Greek yogurt, or can I have half a slice of bread and half a glass of wine?

A Technically, you could do this, but I discourage it—not because I don't want you to have any fun or variety, but because once you start dividing up portions, portion creep happens.

I see this all the time. You have a little more than half a portion of this, a little more than half a portion of that. You stop measuring. You eyeball it. Before you know it, two half portions have turned into two whole portions, and then you're eating Greek yogurt with granola and blueberries and what the heck, some raisins and chocolate chips, too. You see where I'm going with this. You end up cheating yourself. Instead, I prefer you keep it simple and just pick the one thing you want the most. Prioritize and focus.

Q **Can I really have dessert? Is this some kind of a trick?**

A I'm never going to tell you that you can't eat something you really want, whether it's red meat or white flour or coffee or sugar. Even if I know you could have made a more nutritious choice. Yes, you can have cookies or cake or even a doughnut on the 1:1:1 plan! I enjoy the occasional dessert, if I decide that's the carb I want the most. Sometimes I'll have the steak with veggies and then indulge in dessert. As long as it's 1:1:1, it's all good. This is why 1:1:1 is such a powerful strategy: Nothing is off the list and you never feel deprived. This is why you can actually stick with it.

Q **You say I can eat the white flour tortilla or the white bread, but I thought whole grain was better than white flour. Shouldn't I always choose the nutritionally superior foods?**

A Whole grains are more nutrient dense than refined grains, it's true. The more nutrients and fewer calories your food contains, the faster you'll lose weight and the better you'll feel. That's just simple math. Your body needs nutrients, and more nutrient-rich food provides those nutrients more efficiently. So yes, it's good to make the more nutritionally sound choices *most of the time*. But I'm not going to try to guilt you into thinking you should make them *all the time*. People of normal weight enjoy indulgences, and you should be able to, too. Maybe you really want the white-flour tortilla today. Maybe you really want the white rice. However, the more you eat healthful foods, the more you'll learn to prefer whole grains and other nutrient-rich foods more often.

Give your palate a chance to experience new tastes. Be adventurous. But don't give up the things you love, either. Remember, 1:1:1 is about balance, not only in your macronutrients, but in your food choices.

Personally, I prefer the taste of white flour tortillas over the taste of whole wheat tortillas, and although I don't eat a lot of pasta myself, I do love fresh-baked pitas and white basmati rice. But if I do have that delicious, warm pita, maybe wrapped around chicken and fresh veggies with a drizzle of yogurt sauce, I won't have the rice or the dessert in the same meal. As long as your occasional indulgences still adhere to 1:1:1, you'll be fine. And you'll keep losing weight. So enjoy them!

It's all about what you do *most* of the time. You already know

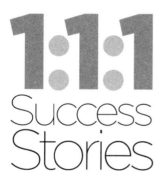

Success Stories

Name: **Amy Ramos**
Starting weight: **189 pounds**
Current weight: **155 pounds**
Height: **4'11"**

I always thought I was healthy. I worked out five to six times a week, went to boot camps, did races, even a half-marathon back in 2010. Looking back, I really wasn't. I still had that "If I work out for an hour I can eat whatever I want" mentality. I was taking in all the calories I burned, and then some. My sister-in-law referred me to Rania about 2 years ago but I didn't contact her for a long time because I was too afraid. What if she wanted me to eat less? Do paleo? Give up desserts? I didn't want that. I'd been on many diets since elementary school—Weight Watchers, Jenny Craig, low-carb, high-carb. You name it, I did it, and I didn't want to do it again.

But I had good reasons to lose weight. In October 2012, the scale said 189, and that was too close to 200 pounds for comfort. I which choices are healthier. I don't have to tell you. You know olive oil is more nutritious than margarine. You know fruit is more nutritious than juice. You know brown rice is more nutritious than white rice. However, you also know what you like. The fact is that variety is more important than always choosing the "perfect" food.

Q I love fruit and I want to be able to eat more fruit, but I've also heard fruit is just as bad for you as sugar. How do I get more fruit without throwing off my ratio?

A Fruit is an excellent carb choice for any meal or snack. It is not "just as bad as sugar" because no food is bad, but it contains

---

also wanted to become a mom and my doctor told me that I had to lose weight before going through in-vitro fertilization. And I wanted to run again. In races with friends, I was always the last one because I was carrying so much weight. I finally got the courage to e-mail Rania, and then we got to work.

The best thing about 1:1:1 is that it doesn't change what I eat. It only changes how and when I eat it. For example, instead of having my sweet potato with chicken for dinner, I swap it for another veggie and have a sweet potato for lunch the next day. I still get my desserts, too—not every night, but I do enjoy them. I didn't have to give them up. Now I have a different outlook on food and how it fuels me, without having to cut out anything. For me, 1:1:1 is all about tweaking what I'm already doing. I've made huge strides in my weight loss journey. I have more self-esteem than I've ever had in my life. I have more energy, I enjoy clothes shopping (a little too much!), and best of all, I'm no longer afraid of wearing a bathing suit. Rania has taught me that "diet" is a four-letter word. Instead, 1:1:1 is a lifestyle change I intend to stick with forever.

more nutrients than pure sugar. However, when you choose it, make it your only carb choice and stick to 1 piece or 1 cup of fruit. To make it more interesting and get more variety, mix it up! Have half a cup of sliced strawberries and half a cup of blueberries, or half a banana mixed with dried raisins and apricots, or a cup of chopped tropical fruit including mango, pineapple, and papaya. Always eat fruit with protein and fat, perhaps by combining pineapple with shredded coconut (fat) and a side of deli ham, or apples with chopped almonds (fat) and a little cheese (protein), and fruit is absolutely fine as a snack or with a meal.

Q Do I have to eat vegetables, salad, or soup with every meal? Can I if I want to?

A You *can* eat these foods at every meal, but only if you want to. Nonstarchy vegetables are free, and you can load up your salad plate or your soup bowl with veggies any time you want, without including them in your 1:1:1 ratio. Just remember that sometimes your meal will be satisfying enough to fill you up on its own. Veggies are a great way to get more fiber and nutrients, so plan them into your diet and prioritize them at mealtime. For example, sneak more veggies into your grains, onto your sandwich, into your omelette, or onto your pizza, or have them as side dishes with dinner.

But again: You don't have to. It's difficult for me to say this as a nutritionist, because I do believe that vegetables and fruits should be a priority in most diets, but so many dieters get caught up in the trap of feeling like they have to cram in more vegetables and fruit all the time, even though they aren't hungry. In fact, many diet plans penned by nutritionists add a salad and fruit to every meal. So many of my clients say they've heard "eat more leafy greens" and "eat more antioxidants" so often that they think these are laws. But they're not laws.

Here's the bottom line: You already know fruit is a carb so it's not an add-on to a meal already containing a carb. Choose it or choose something else, but don't add it to your meal just because you think you should. Vegetables are free, but you don't need to eat them unless you want to. They're a great way to fill up, but not so great if you use them to overstuff yourself in the name of "nutrition."

Stop choking down salads or force-feeding yourself citrus fruits or swallowing vegetable soup to fill you up before your meals when you don't want to. If you're already full from your 1:1:1 meal, you don't need to keep eating. To many of my clients, this is a revelation.

Q But if I don't *have* to eat fruits and vegetables, will I get enough fruits and vegetables? I might never eat them. Don't I need them for good health?

A The 1:1:1 plan puts your health and food choices back into *your* hands, so to some extent, that's up to you. If you get tired of fruits and vegetables, the beauty of 1:1:1 is that you don't have to eat them with every meal. One of the most important parts of 1:1:1 is learning how to eat for yourself, without someone "making you" eat this or that. I want you to feel empowered to make your own food choices. But I'm not above giving you some good reasons to make healthy choices most of the time.

The fact is that vegetables and fruits are full of vitamins, minerals, and fiber, and also low in calories. That's good news for people trying to lose weight. It can be painless to add them, with great benefits—but only when you decide, all by yourself, to choose them.

Q Speaking of salad, a lot of diets tell you to use fat-free dressing, but I think it tastes disgusting, and I'm certainly not going to eat my salad without any dressing. If I use dressing, is that my one fat? Can I put anything fun like feta cheese or sliced almonds or avocados on my salad?

A One of the reasons I love the 1:1:1 plan so much is that it's realistic and rational. I'm not going to ask you to do anything crazy or weird, and I don't ever want you to feel deprived. You get to eat the food you're used to eating. To me, dressing counts as part of the salad. It "comes with" the salad, like shoelaces come with your gym shoes. Try to drizzle your dressing lightly, and remember that olive oil–based dressings are a healthier choice than creamy dressing, but go ahead. Dress those leafy greens, then add one fat on top: cheese or sliced almonds or avocados, if you like them—but just choose one, as your fat serving. Add some salmon (protein) and dried cranberries (carb) and you've got yourself a meal—dressing included.

However, remember that if you're doing 1:1:1 Accelerated, then your dressing should step up and take the place of your fat choice. You can still add salmon and dried cranberries to that salad, but skip the cheese if you want the balsamic vinaigrette.

Q What other foods don't I have to count in my 1:1:1 tally? Are there other "comes with" foods?

A Yes! Here is your list of "comes with" foods on the 1:1:1 plan:
  • Dressing comes with salad.

• Cream or milk comes with coffee or tea (if you like it). Ditto for a teaspoon of sugar.

• Syrup or a little fruit spread comes with your waffle or pancake.

However, remember that if you're on 1:1:1 Accelerated, things change. Dressing is a fat, cream is a fat, syrup is a carb, sugar is a carb, and a serving of bread is one slice, sandwich or no sandwich.

Snack Break

Try this tasty, nutrient-dense snack: Wash a bunch of kale leaves, cut out the thick spines, and tear them into chip-sized pieces. Dry them and toss them with a little bit of olive oil. Spread them on a baking sheet, and roast them for about 15 minutes in a 350°F oven, or until they get crisp. (Watch them carefully—they can burn in a moment!) Remove from the oven, season them with sea salt, and snack on them like potato chips!

Q So wait—I can pretty much be normal, not diet-y?

A Yes! As I said before, 1:1:1 is realistic and rational. If you like cream in your coffee or tea, you should be able to enjoy that and not have to sacrifice the feta in your Greek omelette. French toast isn't a carb and a protein just because it's cooked with an egg. It's a carb. It's French toast. You can still have some turkey sausage on the side.

Honestly, though, although it's traditional, syrup for breakfast along with your carb makes your whole day sloppy. Have you found that when you eat high-carbohydrate breakfasts full of simple sugars, you seem to lose energy and then crave more sweets? But if you always have syrup with your pancakes and you can't imagine pancakes any other way, and you feel okay after eating it, then syrup goes with pancakes. Just remember to balance it out, and you can eat anything, as long as it fits the ratio. That doesn't mean you can't consider doing pancakes (or waffles or French toast) a different way—like spread with almond butter instead of syrup, or dipped into Greek yogurt and cinnamon.

Sometimes people ask me if they can add fruit to their pancakes, and honestly, the answer is no to this one. Fruit doesn't make this dish much healthier—it just makes it a sugar bomb. Save the fruit for your midmorning snack.

Q What about mixed foods, like lasagna or granola? How do you know what they are?

A This is where you use your common sense. A cookie contains butter, but it's a cookie and made mostly with flour and sugar so it's a carb. Granola contains fat and sugar and sometimes dried fruit, but granola is its own thing, so it's a carb. Packaged flavored oatmeal is a thing, so it's a carb, not a double carb. Just don't add fruit!

When it comes to things like casseroles, it can get a little more complicated. Lasagna contains cheese, noodles, and meat, so that's a complete meal—it's 1:1:1. However, if the lasagna is made with mozzarella and ricotta, you count them both as just "cheese" and it's one fat. If it's relatively homogenous, then it is what it is. Just look at it. Step back. What is it? Noodles? Carb. Rice? Carb. Cereal? Carb. Meaty? Protein. Cheesy? Protein or fat. Nutty? Fat. However, if you can clearly discern different elements—like meat, cheese, and crust on a pizza or cereal, fruit, and nuts in a bowl of oatmeal—then count the separate categories. A pizza with pepperoni and cheese is a 1:1:1 meal all by itself. A bowl of oatmeal with walnuts and milk is a 1:1:1 meal all by itself. Use your good judgment. You don't have to spend all day trying to dissect everything you eat. Again, however, remember that things are different on 1:1:1 Accelerated. Take that lasagna. The cheese in the lasagna is a double-doer. It can stand in as a fat and a protein, so choose a veggie lasagna instead of the version with both meat and cheese, which is overdoing it on Accelerated. Veggie lasagna on 1:1:1 Accelerated works out like this: Noodles: carb. Cheese: protein and fat. Veggies: free. If your chili has beans (protein and carb), it doesn't need more protein (like turkey or beef) and you don't need to scoop it up with tortilla chips (more carbs), but some cubed avocado or a spoonful of sour cream would be a fine addition for a fat.

Food for **Thought**

You've probably tried a lot of fruits and vegetables in your life. Think back to some of the fruits and vegetables you've tried in the past—maybe even in childhood—that you loved, or kind of liked, or even hated, but forgot about or haven't had in a long time. Try them again now, and see how your palate has changed. It's fun to be adventurous with your food, and fruits and vegetables are the perfect category in which to engage in some dietary exploration. You might find a new veggie favorite in a childhood veggie nemesis like Brussels sprouts or okra or artichoke!

Q I'm single and I have an active social life. I often go out with my girlfriends and they all drink like guys, but if I have more than two or three drinks, I'm eating everything in sight. How do I moderate my eating and drinking in a social situation?

A No need to cancel girls' night out! Just stick to one drink. After that, ordering water or a club soda will keep you hydrated and also help give your stomach a feeling of fullness so you don't descend on the nacho plate or polish off the Buffalo wings. Remember, even when you're out partying, 1:1:1 is still the goal! Alcohol is a carb, so your food should be protein, veggies, and fat only.

I just had a client come in the other day and decide that one of her goals was to drink no more than one glass of wine for every hour she was out. She calls it her "One Per Hour Rule." In general, I recommend no more than one for the night—your one carb for dinner. However, she knows she's going to drink more, so this is her way to modify it. If you know you're going to cheat when it comes to girls' night out, expect your weight loss to stall for a few days, definitely keep it to one drink per hour, and down plenty of water or club soda between drinks.

Q I really don't eat very much, and 1:1:1 is more than I currently eat. Will I still lose weight?

A If 1:1:1 seems like too much food for you, start with 1:1:1 Accelerated. Also, if you have fewer than 20 pounds to lose, or you've hit a plateau, consider 1:1:1 Accelerated instead of the regular 1:1:1 plan. It's more rigorous, but you'll get faster, more dramatic results. (See Chapter 7.)

Q How often should I weigh myself?

A Everyone is different. Some people like to get a daily weight to help remind them to stay on track, and they find this motivating. For other people, daily weigh-ins are a bad idea because the natural fluctuations of water weight can be distracting and discouraging.

A client of mine says she's more consistent with healthy choices and exercise during the week so she always weighs herself on Wednesdays. She calls them "Weigh-In Wednesdays." This can work for you, too. Pick a day and a time when you think you're at your most representative weight. Whatever it is, always weigh yourself at approximately the same time on the same day for the most accurate idea of your progress.

Q I totally get how 1:1:1 works and I love that I can snack on something like pretzels or chips or even candy if I choose that as my occasional carb. I always buy the large bags because they're much more economical than the smaller portion-sized bags, but my problem is portion control. I want to eat the whole bag! How do I keep myself under control once I start snacking?

A A lot of portion control has to do with packaging. Food companies are smart. They make their packaging exciting and stimulating, so you're triggered to eat more and more. Delicious-looking pictures of the food on the box can also make you grab the box and eat the food, even when you aren't hungry. I recently read a study in the *Journal of Consumer Psychology* that said the picture on the front of a package influences how people think about the product, and people ate more food from packages with many items pictured on them. Don't be fooled! Instead, make things easier on yourself. If you love pretzels or

111

Slim It **Down**

If you love milk chocolate, give dark chocolate a try. Not only does it contain antioxidants, but it's rich and satisfying and has less sugar than white or milk chocolate. Some dark chocolate is even infused with exotic flavors, like citrus peel, cinnamon, raspberry, sea salt, even chile pepper and bacon! What a nice way to add spice to your life.

chips, buy the big bag, which will save you money, but look on the back and see what a serving is. Usually it's about an ounce, or a serving will be indicated as "23 pretzels" or "16 chips." Portion out the whole bag into those little plastic snack bags, label them, and store them in an opaque container in the pantry. Then throw away that tempting, stimulating packaging. When you want a snack, just reach in and grab a bag. There's your serving. Enjoy! By the way, if you've never done this, you'll probably be surprised how satisfying it is. You still get to finish "the whole bag," but it will not add to your saddlebags!

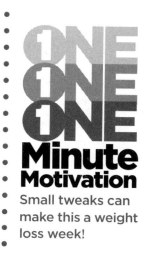

One One One Minute Motivation

Small tweaks can make this a weight loss week!

Q If this is a strategy, why do you call it a diet?

A The 1:1:1 plan is not a diet, in that you don't "go on it" and then "go off it." However, the word diet actually comes from a Latin word that means "a way of life." In that sense, 1:1:1 *is* a diet. It's how you live: in balance.

My main quibble with the word *diet* is when people use it to punish themselves. If there's one thing I can't stand, it's when people think they have to be all diet-y to lose weight. No, you don't! You just have to be sensible. Eating like you're on a diet just makes you feel deprived and irritable. It makes you feel stupid and different and fat—or, on the other hand, superior and self-righteous (until you go home and raid the refrigerator and wallow in guilt). Being on a diet sets you apart from life, and I want you to jump back into life *right now*. And 1:1:1 is your vehicle.

I don't care what the nutritionist or diet book told you. Just because you're overweight doesn't mean you're not allowed to eat like other people. You should be able to get just as much pleasure from your food as a thin person. Sure, your skinny best friend may guzzle margaritas and nachos, but how healthy is that? You can participate in a night out at a Mexican restaurant with all your friends, and you can make choices that don't look any stranger than anyone else's, even though you're following 1:1:1 and choosing not to overdo your carbs. It's something that works in real life. It's *regular eating*.

This is your new life. Your reality check. Your return to sanity. This is how to eat. That's why it's a strategy. Really, 1:1:1 is a lifestyle—and a choice you've made—to get back into balance, regain your health, and achieve the weight your body was meant to be.

CHAPTER NINE

Eating Out with 1:1:1

W hy don't regular diets let you have any fun? It's not fair, is it? People who are trying to lose weight often think they can never go out to eat. Restaurants are danger zones! They have bread baskets and chip baskets and giant portions full of fat, salt, and sugar! They have appetizers and cocktails and desserts! It's a dieter's nightmare!

You can calm down. This all may be true, but if you're eating according to 1:1:1, then you're not technically a "dieter." You're not following anyone's meal plan. You're choosing your own foods and strategically moderating your intake. That means you don't have to worry about restaurants, thank goodness. You can go out and have fun whenever you want to, and order whatever you want. The only thing you have to keep in mind is 1:1:1.

Let me repeat: *You can have whatever you want at a restaurant.* This may sound counterintuitive, especially for people who have been dieting for years. One of my clients told me that when she's trying to lose weight, she orders tacos without the cheese and sour cream. All her tacos contain are meat and lettuce. She's got the carb (the shell) and the protein (the meat) but no fat, so the taco isn't likely to keep her full for very long, nor to satisfy her in the short term because she admitted she doesn't even really like tacos that way. She orders them without the cheese and sour cream because she thinks that's a sacrifice you have to make if you want your diet to work. I set her straight. You don't have to give up every single decadent-sounding food you love. Eat what you really want to eat, but choose the cheese *or* the sour cream, to add fat to your meal, put it back into balance, *and* make it more pleasurable to eat. Otherwise, you're probably just going to be looking for something to eat later because that dry tortilla shell with a little bit of chicken and lettuce in it didn't satisfy your appetite or your tastebuds.

Here's another rule you can break for good: So many diet books recommend that you ask for a "doggie bag" when you order your meal and put half of it in the container to take home *before you even start eating.* That's ridiculous. Who really does that, except someone being all diet-y? Normal people don't freak out about how much they might eat before they've even gotten started. Order according to 1:1:1, and if you're hungry enough to eat it all, then just eat it all. You're in a restaurant. You're paying a lot for that food, so enjoy it. Sure, if they pile your plate with a mountain of pasta, notice that. Pay attention to how you feel as you eat and eat until you're just pleasantly satisfied, not stuffed to the gills. Remind yourself that you'll feel better later if you do. It's important to notice when you're getting too full and stop eating. *Then* you can ask for a to-go box and take the rest home for lunch tomorrow. That's how "normal people" eat. And you know what else? I don't care how they prepared your food in the kitchen. If you hate some ingredient or can't eat some ingredient because of a health problem, sure, ask about it and make sure they don't put what you don't want in your food. But you don't have to grill the waiter about how the cook grilled the food. Is that butter? Olive oil? Is it light? Heavy? Is there cream? Is the dressing on the side?

Stop it. Just eat what you want and order what you want and forget about all the embarrassing diet-y things you think you're supposed to do and say and ask for. Order according to 1:1:1, then just eat your food, enjoy it, and be satisfied. If you want more veggies instead of the blue cheese potato or rice pilaf because you know you want a glass of wine, simply order what you want. Skip the bread basket, but don't talk about it—just do it! Talking about it makes you focus on it more, and then you feel deprived, and then you eat it anyway, even if it really isn't all that good.

I know how hard this is to grasp if you've been dieting for years. Order anything you want? The very idea of a restaurant feels overwhelming. Even when you have a handle on 1:1:1 at home, staying on track at a restaurant can seem a little scary. My clients often tell me they get nervous about going out with friends, especially the ones who tend to overeat or who will definitely order dessert. (You know what I'm talking about—you probably have friends like that, too.) They think they won't be able to enjoy their favorite dishes on the menu anymore. They worry about going on dates and feeling pressured to get an appetizer and a big entrée and too many drinks. They don't want to look like they're dieting, but they don't want to feel so anxious that they end up obsessing over the food and forget to enjoy themselves. Or they have to eat out a lot for work and don't know how they're supposed to do that without blowing their diet.

I don't want my clients—or you—to feel like they can't live normal lives, and part of normal life is going out to eat! It shouldn't be such a big deal. It's just going out to eat. It doesn't have to have so much anxiety attached to it. Eating should be fun, and socializing while eating makes it even more fun. You don't have to give that up at all, as long as you pay

Food for **Thought**

Never "save up" your calories for a restaurant meal by skipping a meal or snack or skimping on protein, carbs, or fat earlier in the day. Stay in balance! It's the best way to make sure you don't overeat when eating out.

attention to what you're doing and keep your meals in line with 1:1:1. Luckily, that's easy to do.

In this chapter, I'll give you ideas for how to order according to 1:1:1 at all sorts of different styles of restaurants. If you're on 1:1:1 Accelerated, I've got suggestions for you, too. (I really mean it when I say anyone can eat at a restaurant!) Every restaurant will have many possibilities, so don't be afraid! Go on—get all dressed up and go! You've been looking particularly slim lately.

1:1:1 Restaurant Strategies

When you go to a restaurant, you can eat what you normally eat. It's just about deciding which menu item you want on this particular visit. Remember, this is not your first trip to a restaurant, and it won't be your last. Some things to remember:

- **Don't show up hungry.** If you arrive at the restaurant starving, you're going to dive into the bread basket and never come out. Do not skip your afternoon snack. I never want you to, but it's especially important when you're going out for dinner. You can be pleasantly hungry but you should never be ravenous.

- **Check out the menu online.** Most restaurants have the menu available online. Read everything over so you can plan what to order ahead of time. This takes the pressure off. You won't have to make a rush decision when the server appears at the table and you've been deep in conversation and haven't figured out which 1:1:1 food combination you want to try that night. Be ready to go and, no matter how nervous or excited you are when you get to the restaurant, you'll be calm, cool, and collected when you order your food.

- **You can have an appetizer.** If you're on a date or out with a friend and your friend wants to split an appetizer, or you want one of your own, you can say yes! However, realize that the shrimp cocktail or the chicken satay skewers are your protein, so don't get the filet mignon for your entrée. Choose pasta primavera or vegetable risotto instead (remember to notice when you've eaten enough). If the appetizer is fries or chips and salsa, that's your carb. Your dinner can be salmon and vegetables or a big salad with grilled chicken. And remember a vegtable soup or a vegetable salad can serve as an appetizer and they are free foods.

- **You can have dessert.** If you're out with the girls who always want dessert, have dessert! Just know that's your carb, so you'll say no thanks to the bread and the pasta and cocktails. Also consider that restaurant dessert portions are probably pretty hefty, and maybe suggest you all split something. Friends share, right?

- **You can have a glass of wine** . . . or a beer or a cocktail. Just make it your carb. Enjoy every sip, and order salad with chicken or fish, or a nice piece of meat with grilled vegetables for dinner. One of my favorite strategies to suggest to my clients is to have your wine or cocktail after the meal. This accomplishes several goals: It can feel like dessert, so you won't feel the need for dessert. You'll get to focus totally on it, which you may not do if you're sipping it with your food. (I suggest drinking water with your meal, to hydrate you pre-cocktail.) And, you'll already be full, so it's the best time to exercise control. (Drinking before your meal can actually stimulate your appetite.)

- **Restaurants do serve 1:1:1 Accelerated-appropriate fare.** If you're on the Accelerated plan, just remember that your carb is vegetables, so choose a protein- and veggie-heavy meal, like shrimp salad or salmon with grilled veggies. Or make your restaurant night your "cheat night," or your one night for alcohol or dessert, but remember that 1:1:1 still applies!

- **You always have choices!** Remember that you are not deprived. You get to choose which protein you want, which carb you want, which fat you want. And the next time you go to a restaurant (or have any meal), you'll get to choose all over again. Freedom!

OK, now that we've gotten the basics out of the way, let's take a culinary world tour, 1:1:1 style.

American/Steakhouse

Steakhouses have a lot of great choices. You aren't going to have trouble in the protein department! They usually serve a variety of vegetables and salads, too, so you can bulk up your meal for free. But you might have some difficulty decoding the tempting side dishes like twice-baked potatoes (carb and fat) or macaroni and cheese (carb and fat) or creamed spinach (vegetable and fat). Here are some of my favorite steakhouse meals and ways to work in those sides, if you want them.

Option 1: Filet mignon (protein), twice-baked potato or baked potato

111 Slim It **Down**

Maybe you're crazy for croutons, and if you are, fine. But if you don't really care about croutons, you might want to leave them off your salad and save your carb choice for something more interesting—because croutons count!

In fact, a lot of carbs that you might not notice count. For example: **Crackers with your soup.** That's your carb, so if your soup has noodles, rice, or potatoes in it, you're double-dipping. Nix the crackers or get soup sans starch.

Chips and salsa. Do you want to have your carb before dinner even starts, or would you rather save it for a burrito, enchilada, or margarita?

The bread basket. You might be hungry now, but have some water and wait for your food. Bread basket bread isn't usually very good. Or ask friends whether it's worth your carb, and if it is, enjoy it!

Since carbs in particular are the most difficult category for people to limit, and a likely contributor to weight problems for many, you might as well not have them when they don't matter that much.

with sour cream or butter and chives (carb and fat), steamed broccoli (free) (optional add: side salad)

Option 2: Pan-seared oysters (protein), creamed spinach (fat), Caesar salad (free), glass of white wine (carb)

Option 3: Grilled chicken breast (protein) with creamy mushroom sauce (fat), risotto (carb), tomato/onion salad (free)

Accelerated dinner option: Salmon filet or sirloin steak (protein), veggie mix or broccoli (carb), house salad with balsamic vinaigrette (fat)

Italian Restaurant

You're already thinking pasta, right? It's the most popular dish at Italian restaurants, and it can be your carb if you love it. Add some meat or seafood for your protein and some cheese, creamy sauce, or butter- or oil-based sauce for your fat. You could also have pasta with chicken, olive oil, garlic, and a green veggie (like broccoli rabe, broccoli, spinach, or asparagus). Or begin your meal with meat antipasto (protein) and order cheese ravioli (fat from cheese, carb from the pasta) with marinara sauce (free because it's made from vegetables). However, pasta isn't the only Italian option. Here are some other choices to consider.

Option 1: Minestrone soup (protein from beans, carb from pasta, free vegetables) topped with Parmesan cheese (fat) (optional add: side of green beans or side salad)

Option 2: Calamari (protein) with a Caprese salad with tomatoes (free), mozzarella cheese (fat), and fresh basil (free), and a glass of Chianti (carb) (optional add: asparagus)

Option 3: Veal Parmesan (protein from veal, fat from cheese), risotto (carb), sautéed zucchini (free) (optional add: side salad)

Accelerated dinner option: Meatballs (protein) in marinara sauce (free), hold the pasta, with grilled zucchini (carb) and a side salad with Italian dressing (fat).

Mexican Restaurant

Mexican restaurants are carb heaven. It's tempting to nosh on the tortilla chips with salsa while sipping a couple of margaritas and then

①①①

Slim It **Down**

Love salsa, but don't want the accompanying chips to be your carb?
Order it! Salsa (or pico de gallo) is a vegetable, so it's a free food.
You can use it to top your burrito or put it on a salad to have as an
appetizer. In fact, shredded lettuce is a common side at Mexican
restaurants. Topped with a little salsa, it's crunchy and satisfying.
Who needs the chips?

---

get the enchiladas or the burrito, with beans and rice nestled in a flour
or corn tortilla—but that's already five carbs! The good news is that
you can have any carb you choose—even if it's flan or fried ice cream
for dessert! Just pick the one you want, and save the others for future
visits. Here are some muy bueno ways to practice 1:1:1 at Mexican
restaurants.

Option 1: Chicken taco salad (protein) with guacamole (fat); skip the
taco shell and have a margarita (carb)

Option 2: Beef, chicken, or bean (protein) burrito (hold the rice, the
tortilla is your carb), with shredded cheese (fat), side of lettuce with salsa
as a dressing (free)

Option 3: Fish (protein) tacos (tortillas are your carb) with avocado
slices (fat)

Accelerated dinner option: Beef, chicken, or shrimp (protein) fajitas
with lots of grilled veggies (carb) and guacamole (fat). Hold the tortillas—
just eat with a fork—delicious!

Japanese Restaurant

Japanese restaurants appear to be full of healthful options, and they
are—but it's also easy to overdo it. Think about a sushi roll: Many are
1:1:1 by themselves, if they contain fish (protein), rice (carb), and

avocado, mayonnaise, or fried "crunchies" (fat). Add edamame, hand rolls, nigiri, and it's way too much.

However, there are plenty of ways to eat until you're full and stick to 1:1:1 at a Japanese restaurant. For one thing, miso soup, seaweed or wakame salad, and lettuce salad are free. (Edamame, on the other hand, is a protein, so pass on it unless you plan to get veggie sushi rolls or vegetable tempura.)

If you go to a Teppanyaki grill—you know, those restaurants where they cook your meal in front of you and do tricks!—you can get any meat (chicken, beef, seafood is your protein) with fried rice (carb), sauce (fat), and a side salad (free). You don't also need sushi. Here are some more ideas.

Option 1: If you're dining with a group and they want to order a bunch of different rolls, try them all, as long as you don't have more than 8 or 10 pieces (the equivalent of what's in one good-sized sushi roll). Most sushi rolls are 1:1:1, with fish (protein), rice (carb), avocado or mayo or crunch (fat), and seaweed and vegetables (free). (Optional add: miso soup)

Option 2: A big bowl of meat or seafood soup (protein) and noodles (carb), or get the soup with no noodles and have sake or a beer (carb) and a side of avocado (fat)

Option 3: Seafood or chicken (protein) tempura (the batter is your carb) and a side salad with avocado (fat)

Accelerated dinner option: Sashimi (protein) with seaweed or wakame salad (veggies are your carb, dressing is your fat). Have miso soup, too, if you need something more.

Chinese Restaurant

Chinese food is a quick option for take-out and it can also be an upscale dining experience. Either way, the sauce on most Chinese dishes counts as your fat because that's mostly what it's made of. Watch out for fried appetizers with dough, like egg rolls and wontons—those count as your carb and if you choose them, you need to skip the rice. There are some free items at a Chinese restaurant, however—hot and sour soup and steamed vegetables. Here are some 1:1:1 ordering ideas when you go Chinese.

Option 1: Chicken egg roll (chicken is your protein, wrapper is your carb) and egg drop soup (fat)

Option 2: Steamed pork dumplings (protein and carb), any stir-fry vegetable entrée (free) with your favorite sauce, like brown or Szechuan (fat)

Option 3: Sweet and sour chicken (sauce is fat, chicken is protein) with rice (carb)

Accelerated dinner option: Any stir-fried entrée with meat (protein), sauce (fat), and vegetables (carb), including nuts (fat), such as cashew chicken, or beef and broccoli or Szechuan shrimp. Hold the rice. If you want more food, add hot and sour soup.

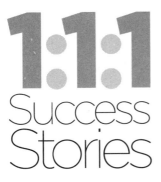

1:1:1 Success Stories

Name: **Barrie Cowan**
Starting weight: **252 pounds**
Current weight: **207 pounds**
Height: **6'2"**

When I was about 50 years old, I was hiking on a steep hillside and fell. I had a lot of trouble getting up, and that scared me. Shortly afterwards, I saw a photograph of myself and realized I looked just like my mother, who was never able to overcome her obesity. Vanity, embarrassment, and fear about my future health spurred me to make a change. Another not insignificant motivation: My wife was concerned about my well-being and I wanted to look good for her! I contacted Rania and she helped me see that I was eating too many carbs and showed me how to balance them with 1:1:1. For example, when I got soup for lunch, I did not take the chunk of French bread that came with it. When I got a sandwich, I

Indian Restaurant

The number-one decision to make at an Indian restaurant: Choose either the rice or the naan, but not both. Also, many Indian dishes have a lot of oil and/or butter in their sauces, so these count as your fat. Unless you want to spend your carb portion at the beginning of the meal and stick to meat and vegetables for your entrée, avoid the batter-fried appetizers like samosas and pakora.

Option 1: Chicken biryani (chicken is protein, sauce is the fat) with basmati rice (carb)

Option 2: Saag paneer (cheese is the protein, spinach is free) with buttered naan (fat and carb)

Option 3: Any vegetarian dish with potatoes, like aloo gobi (potatoes

---

didn't get the little bag of potato chips. I stopped going to the Japanese udon noodle place and similar carb-heavy lunch spots and changed my afternoon pick-me-up snack to one small, healthy nutrition bar or a piece of fruit with some protein. I stopped eating desserts at home and I ate out less often, which helped me to practice 1:1:1 under more controlled conditions. I never felt like I was on a diet—I felt like I was the one in charge of my choices, so I had a feeling of moral satisfaction in the beginning. As the weight loss became substantial—I lost about 25 pounds in the first couple of months—I was restored to a level of strength and fitness I hadn't even realized I had lost. I began to feel very good about myself. The 1:1:1 method helped me to find a balance among the internal forces contending for my conscious attention, so that I was finally able to hear the natural—but often very quiet—inward voice of moderation and purpose in eating. My results have been quite stable over the past two and a half years, and I am now down 45 pounds!

are the carb, sauce is the fat) with a skewer of lamb or chicken (protein)

Accelerated dinner option: Tandoori chicken (protein) with a cucumber salad (carb) and yogurt dressing (fat), or any curry (sauce is the fat) with meat (protein) and vegetables (carb), hold the rice and the naan

Mediterranean Restaurant

Tabouli, hummus, stuffed grape leaves—to me, this is comfort food. My family is from the Middle East and this is the cuisine I grew up eating. I just love it but not only because I'm familiar with it: It's also a cuisine that's very compatible with 1:1:1, with many dishes naturally balancing a protein with a carb and a fat, along with a lot of vegetables. There are many carb choices in Mediterranean food—pita, rice, tabouli—but of course, you'll pick the one you want the most. Some ideas (I can't help adding an extra option to this category):

Option 1: Gyro (the lamb or other meat is your protein, pita is your carb, yogurt sauce is your fat, and veggies are free). Add a side salad if you need more.

Option 2: Sumac chicken (protein) and fattoush salad (the Mediterranean version of Caesar salad, with pita instead of croutons for your carb) topped with feta cheese (fat)

Option 3: Tabouli salad (bulgur wheat is your carb) with hummus (protein) drizzled with a little olive oil (fat)

Option 4: Dolmades, also called stuffed grape leaves, filled with ground meat (protein) and rice (carb), tomatoes and cucumber salad (free), and topped with feta cheese (fat)

Accelerated dinner option: Kebab (use any meat for your protein, like lamb or chicken) with babaghanoush (eggplant is your carb, tahini is your fat)

Buffet

It's all too easy to go overboard at a buffet. There are so many choices and you have the opportunity to revisit the food again and again. But with 1:1:1, you can make smart choices and enjoy yourself. The options here are designed not only to be balanced but also to help you check the temptation to pile your plate high with everything available.

Before you begin, take a walk around the entire buffet to see what looks good, so you can decide which things you really want the most. Wouldn't you hate to choose macaroni and cheese before you see the dessert bar, or settle for soggy French fries before noticing that fresh garlic bread?

Option 1: Head to the carving station. Get a nice slice of roasted meat (protein), then fill your plate with green beans, Brussels sprouts, cooked spinach (free). Add a scoop of mashed potatoes (carb) with gravy (fat), and you're good to go!

Option 2: If you like the look of a mixed dish, like lasagna, chicken teriyaki, or frittata, that's just fine, but pay attention to what it contains. Lasagna has noodles (carb), meat (protein), and fat (cheese). Chicken teriyaki has meat (protein) and sauce (fat), and you can add rice for your carb. Frittata contains egg (protein) and veggies (free), and cheese (fat). Have a croissant on the side as your carb. Just pick the one thing you want, pay attention to what it contains, and enjoy it! This is a more satisfying and sensible option than choosing a little bit of everything and losing track of how much you're eating. Add a salad if you want more bulk.

Option 3: If the buffet has to-die-for desserts, then have a salad with some protein only, and save your carb for the sweet treat that looks the best. The same goes for mimosas or Bloody Marys. If you choose an alcoholic drink, that's your carb.

Option 4: If it's a breakfast buffet, the omelet station is probably your best bet. Get an omelet (eggs are your protein) with cheese (fat) and lots of yummy veggies (free). Add toast, hash browns, *or* fruit—but only one (carb).

Accelerated dinner option: Go wild at the salad station, choosing as many veggies (carb) as you can. Add chicken or chickpeas (protein), and either use dressing or dress your salad with a scoop of something creamy like coleslaw (fat). (Skip the carb choices like fruit, crackers, and macaroni or potato salad.) The great thing about salad bars is you can really pile your plate high, and still stay in balance. If you go back for seconds, make sure it's only for veggies.

Coffeehouse

Most diets tell you to stop drinking coffee, but why be miserable? A lot of people refuse to follow a diet plan that requires them to give up coffee, and I don't blame them. Coffee is comforting, exhilarating, and such a common habit that the country would probably collapse if it was all taken away. It's also the number-one source of antioxidants consumed worldwide.

Even though cream or milk "comes with" coffee on the 1:1:1 plan, we all know big sugary lattes with whole milk and sugar syrup and whipped cream are excessive. If you really want to slim it down and make room for more nutritious food choices, try getting used to drinking regular black coffee. (Definitely do this if you are on 1:1:1 Accelerated and want your fat in some other form.) Coffeehouses often feature delicious flavored coffee beans and different roasts, which you can taste better if the coffee is black. (The flavor in coffee, like vanilla, is infused into the bean. They don't contain sugar.) One cup of black coffee with breakfast is fine, and free (a splash of milk or cream goes with it, if you like it better that way). With black coffee, you'll get a nice energy boost and you may be less likely to indulge in cup after cup because it doesn't contain appetite-stimulating sugar. This is important because too much caffeine can disrupt the blood sugar/insulin cycle in some people. It can also tax your adrenal glands, aggravate stress, contribute to poor sleep quality, and even cause abnormal heart rhythms in some people, so why go overboard? Coffee in moderation is linked to better health, but that's one or two cups a day. If you plan to be hanging around reading or working in the coffeehouse all day, you can still drink cup after cup—just switch to herbal tea after one or two cups of joe. Try a seasonal flavor or something relaxing like chamomile or rejuvenating like peppermint.

Here are some ideas about what to order, to stay in balance the next time you're visiting a Starbucks or your local, hip coffeehouse.

Option 1: Breakfast sandwich with bread (carb), egg (protein), and cheese (fat), with a black coffee (free, even if you add a splash of milk)

Option 2: Small muffin (carb) with butter (fat), latte with fat-free milk (protein)

Option 3: Turkey (protein) and avocado (fat) on a baguette (carb) with herbal tea. Vegetarian option: Caprese sandwich (mozzarella is your protein; the bread is your carb) with pesto spread (fat) and green tea or red Rooibos.

Option 4: Packet of almonds (fat) with a vanilla latte or hot chocolate (carb and protein)

Accelerated dinner option: Have a salad (carb) with chicken or tuna (protein) and tea or coffee with cream (fat).

Fast Food

There's nothing inherently wrong with fast food. An occasional cheeseburger or order of fries or even a milk shake isn't going to kill you or make you fat. Like everything else, you just need to eat it in balance. If you want soda, don't have a bun with your burger or fries, because you chose your carb. If you want the fries, drink water and try a salad with chicken. If you want a good old-fashioned cheeseburger, that's 1:1:1 all by itself, so you don't need fries or a soda. The burger is your protein, the bun is your carb, and the cheese is your fat (or skip the cheese and add bacon, or skip the bacon and add mayonnaise). Other suggestions:

Option 1: Chili (meat is protein, beans are carb) with shredded cheese or sour cream (fat) (if you need more, have a side salad)

Option 2: Chicken sandwich (chicken is protein, bun is carb) with mayo (fat) and a side salad

Option 3: Small fries (carb), cheeseburger (meat is protein, cheese is fat) without the bun, served with lettuce and tomato (free)

Option 4: Small milk shake (carb), grilled chicken salad with cheese (chicken is protein, cheese is fat)

Option 5: Baked potato (carb) with broccoli (free), cheese (protein), and sour cream (fat)

Option 6: A 6-inch sub sandwich (the bread is your carb) with meat (protein), cheese or mayonnaise (fat), and all the veggies you want (free).

Note: A 6-inch sub is a full meal. A 12-inch sub is two meals. If you can't resist the 12-inch, enjoy half for lunch and save the other half for your midafternoon snack, or tomorrow's lunch.

Breakfast option 1: Sausage patty (protein), scrambled egg (fat), hash browns (carb)

Breakfast option 2: Breakfast sandwich made with bacon or egg (protein), cheese (fat), and English muffin or croissant (carb), black coffee

Accelerated dinner option: Any fast food salad (meat is protein, vegetables are the carb, hold the croutons or tortilla strips) with dressing (fat). (If this is lunch, you can add a starchy carb like croutons, crackers, potato chips, dried fruit, or sweet potato fries.)

I hope this convinces you that you'll never have to be afraid to eat at a restaurant again. Social plans: officially back on!

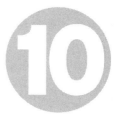

CHAPTER TEN

Working Out with 1:1:1

E xercise is good. This isn't a revelation, right? You already know you're supposed to exercise. You might also already know the benefits of exercise, but just in case you need a little reminder:

- Exercise burns fat and it builds muscle, which burns more fat even when you're just lying on the couch watching the latest dance- or fitness-based reality show.

- Exercise keeps your heart healthier, so you're less likely to have a heart attack.

- Exercise lowers blood pressure, which also helps prevent heart disease.

- Exercise just makes you feel better. It improves your mood as well as antidepressants, according to one study. And it improves self-esteem.

- Moderate exercise might help motivate you to stick to healthy eating. (Extreme exercise is likely to make you hungrier.) Comfort food may give you a boost of feel-good endorphins, but so does exercise! If you exercise, you won't crave that comfort food as much. (Although you may feel like you need to eat more to compensate for that extra calorie burn, you're likely to make healthier choices.)

- Exercise gives you more energy, so the more you exercise, the more you feel like exercising, as well as doing everything else—like cooking dinner, walking the dog, or auditioning for that reality show you've been watching.

- Exercise makes you look better. It's okay to be a little vain—who doesn't want a glowing complexion, not to mention tighter arms, flatter abs, more shapely legs, and a great butt?

- Exercise boosts your sex drive. You might end up having more sex—which is more exercise!

There is no doubt that exercise has superpowers. One of my clients says that when she works out, her reactions to others are more civil and she can better tolerate the little irritations in life! Without it, she says she feels guilty and moody and eats too much chocolate after dinner but doesn't even enjoy it because she feels out of control.

To me, actually being able to enjoy eating chocolate is reason enough to exercise! And if exercise can help you feel calmer and less irritable while also making you look better and feel stronger and more energetic, well . . . it's hard to argue against it.

There is, however, one thing exercise might not do: Just on its own, it probably won't help you lose weight in the long term.

People are often surprised by this, but the truth is, dietary changes—not activity—are mostly responsible for weight loss. Study after study has

Start-Now Strategy

So you haven't exercised for a while? No problem. You can take it one day at a time. Today, head outside and go for a 15-minute walk. It's only 15 minutes—you waste that much time Googling things you don't even care that much about!

shown that dietary changes are more powerful indicators of weight loss than exercise, although exercise can support and enhance this effect. "But I work out like crazy! Why can't I lose weight?" my clients ask all the time. The answer almost always is (sorry), you're eating too much or eating out of balance. Despite what you may think, exercise doesn't give you a free pass to eat anything any where, any time.

Exercise does rev up your appetite. If you don't change what and how you eat, exercise will give you stronger muscles and a healthier heart, but maybe not a smaller waistline. If your postworkout hunger rages out of control, as it does for some people, then you might even gain weight.

Exercise also has its risks. If you overdo it, trying to maximize that calorie burn, you'll be more prone to injury. If you get hurt, it can stop your exercise regimen cold. When you stop exercising, the pounds pile on fast if your diet is not up to par. This happened to one of my clients, Bill. He had a crappy diet (his words!) but managed to lose 40 pounds by doing 2-hour workouts 5 days a week. Then he blew out his knee and, other than physical therapy, was not active at all. He put on all the weight he lost and then some, gaining 50 pounds. So much for the weight loss power of his exercise routine!

However, the good news is that there is a highly effective middle ground—a way to get all the benefits of exercise *and* boost your weight loss: If you eat according to 1:1:1, *and also exercise,* then exercise *can* help you lose weight. You won't be eating more in response to exercise because your meals and portions are already under control.

I like to get my clients secure with the 1:1:1 plan before we even talk about changing what they do for exercise. I don't want them to be shaky or prone to cheating due to excessive hunger. I want them to really understand how great 1:1:1 makes them feel. *Then* we talk about how they can boost their weight loss even more with exercise.

Balanced exercise, that is.

Balancing your exercise means getting not too little, but not too much, and not all one type of exercise either. This may not be what you're doing now, even if you exercise regularly. Just as people tend to eat what they like, people tend to exercise the way they like. Cardio people may run to the gym, run at the gym, and run home but never do anything else. Yoga people may take several classes a week but rarely get their heart rates up. And weight-training people with impressive muscles may barely be able to touch their knees, let alone their toes, or those muscles may be covered by a stubborn layer of fat they never try to burn off with cardio.

If you tend to do only one thing—if you tend to be a cardio person or a yoga person or a weight-lifting person—you could be exercising better and smarter than you are right now.

You could be exercising according to 1:1:1.

Exercise Imbalance

I see exercise imbalance in my clients all the time. I have one client, JoAnn, who does constant cardio but no resistance training or stretching. She took up running specifically for the purpose of losing weight. She knew a lot of "skinny runners," and she wanted to be one of them.

JoAnn is dedicated—she runs about 5 miles on most days, and she races. I can't even imagine doing this! She loves it. Yet she was still about 20 pounds overweight and couldn't figure out why.

When I looked at JoAnn's food diary, the answer was clear to me. She was eating a lot of carbs and fat, but not enough protein. She's been

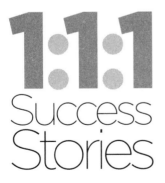

Name: **Jane Costello**
Starting weight: **243 pounds**
Current weight: **168 pounds**
Height: **5′9″**

I had struggled with my weight all my life, and in my late twenties I was officially obese. I was so desperate to lose weight that I met with a bariatric surgeon to discuss lap band surgery. My insurance required that I have supervised weight loss for 6 months before it would pay for the operation. Rania and I met in September 2011 running for years, but she has no upper body strength and I suspect a chronic protein deficiency has led to muscle breakdown. She's out of balance, but her routine feels balanced to her because she's used to it. Nevertheless, those 20 extra pounds are proof that something isn't working.

JoAnn's favorite post-running snack is peanut butter. Great, except for the fact that her idea of a serving is 6 tablespoons! That's about 600 calories and 48 grams of fat, for a snack! A more balanced choice: 1 tablespoon of PB spread on apple slices with a glass of milk. I also suggested she alternate running with another form of exercise, for a more balanced approach. She's "looking into" a yoga class, and has meanwhile cut back on the peanut butter. Now she's losing some weight—5 pounds in the first 2 weeks!

On the opposite side of the spectrum, we have Susan, my client who only does yoga and meditation. She's very calm, but she has no muscle tone and gets winded going up a flight of stairs. Because she doesn't have a lot of muscle, she isn't burning as much fat as she could be while at rest, and her cardiovascular fitness is abysmal. She was surprised when I told her that yoga wasn't enough to keep her balanced, fitness wise.

"But I thought yoga did everything!" she said.

Yoga is good for you. It involves stretching and even an element of

and she helped me find balance in my diet. With her 1:1:1 approach, I lost 25 pounds in 2 months. I was feeling so good that I decided to try a boot camp class. It was hard and I hated it at first, but gradually I grew to love it—especially when I started losing even more weight. I lost an additional 40 pounds after that by combining 1:1:1 Accelerated and exercise, for a total of 75 pounds so far! Needless to say, I cancelled my lap band surgery. This is still a journey for me, but now I know that I can do it on my own, using 1:1:1 and exercising most days of the week! People ask me every day how I lost the weight, and I always tell them: I learned how to eat in balance, and I reclaimed my inner athlete!

resistance training because you have to lift your own body weight in some of the poses. Some active forms can also serve as a cardio workout, if they are flow styles where you move continuously and work up a sweat. However, Susan practiced a style that's very focused on stretching and relaxing. That's fine, especially since stress can make losing weight much harder (see the next chapter), but it doesn't burn calories. Yoga is most effective for weight loss and maintenance if you balance it with other types of exercise.

Now I have Susan doing 20 minutes of cardio and 20 minutes of resistance training using light weights just 3 days a week, in addition to her regular yoga classes. She not only looks better, with a body more in proportion, but those 10 pounds she wants to lose are finally peeling off—and she has more energy. "I ran up the stairs yesterday!" she told me on our last call.

One of my male clients, Tom, is a weight lifter. He drinks high-calorie protein shakes because he wants to gain more muscle, but he's very thick and he keeps getting thicker—so thick that it's hard to see any muscle definition beneath the layers of body fat. He's a big guy and very strong, but he's not "ripped" or "cut" or "shredded" (or whatever the kids call it these days!). Plus, he can't even begin to touch his toes. He's muscle-bound and overweight.

Tom was very attached to his routine, so first I had to convince him that his protein shake was a complete meal, not an add-on. He'd been having it along with his breakfast. I asked him to bring in the shake mix so we could look at it together, and I showed him that it contained a lot of great protein, but also a high dose of carbs (it was sweetened) and enough fat for a meal. It was a 1:1:1 all by itself, so it didn't need any additions—not fruit, not yogurt, not raw eggs, and definitely not a side of bacon or a hunk of Cheddar cheese.

Tom argued that fruit, yogurt, and eggs are all healthy foods, and I agreed! I explained that if Tom wanted to have eggs (protein), cheese (fat), and fruit (carb) or Greek yogurt (protein), fruit (carb), and nuts (fat) for breakfast, he could certainly do that, but then he had to save the protein shake for another meal—or have it as a snack.

Once we got his diet in balance and he was using the protein shakes appropriately, I brought up the topic of cardio. He hated running and couldn't imagine himself in an exercise class, but one of the guys he knew from the gym was a Spinning instructor, so he agreed to try a class. He loved it! It felt natural and he liked the music the instructor played during the class. Spinning fuels his competitive nature, and he's learning how to push himself and work up a sweat, outside the weight room. Now we're finally starting to see steady weight loss. Next step: getting him to try a yoga class. (One step at a time . . . this can be your approach, too!)

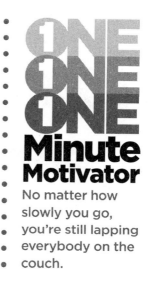

ONE ONE ONE Minute Motivator

No matter how slowly you go, you're still lapping everybody on the couch.

Balancing Exercise with 1:1:1

Maybe you saw this coming . . . but you can apply 1:1:1 to exercise in much the same way you apply it to your diet! A well-rounded exercise program adheres to 1:1:1 because it includes equal parts of these very important types of exercise.

- Cardiovascular exercise or "cardio" (like running, biking, brisk walking, or using the elliptical trainer or rowing machine at the gym)

- Strength or resistance training (like weight lifting on your own with free weights or weight machines, or certain kinds of exercise classes)

- Stretching and relaxation (like yoga, or any kind of stretching class, as well as things like meditation that calm you)

Just as you need to know which foods are primarily made of carbs, proteins, and fats, you also need to know which exercises fall under each category: cardio, strength or resistance, and stretching. This can be confusing because some exercises, and especially exercise classes, combine two or three. An aerobics class might start with cardio, do some strength training (like floor exercises), and end with stretching and relaxation. Classes like these are exercise double-doers (or even triple-doers). They count for more than one category.

There are a lot of activities you can do so I'm probably leaving some things out, but in general, this is how I classify the different types of exercise.

Cardio	Strength/ Resistance	Stretching/ Relaxing
Brisk walking or running, swimming, active outdoor sports like cycling, skating, or skiing	Free weights, like barbells and dumbbells, or weight machines	The types of yoga focused on alignment and stretching, like Iyengar yoga
Cardio machines like elliptical trainers, treadmills, rowing machines, and stationary bicycles	Hydraulic or pneumatic resistance machines	Slow, meditative styles of yoga that hold positions for a long time or focus on relaxation, like restorative, Kripalu, or Yin yoga
Step aerobics, BodyStep, and other aerobics-style classes, either at a gym or on DVD	Pilates, especially classes that use the reformer machine (but mat classes also build strength)	Slow walks out in nature
Dance fitness classes like ballet, barre, ballroom dancing, and hip-hop, including dance fitness classes like Zumba and Be Moved	Calisthenics that make you lift your own body weight, like pushups, crunches, squats, and lunges	Gentle stretching you do on your own at home
Kickboxing and other martial arts classes	Exercises using kettlebells, medicine balls, or heavy ropes	Relaxation classes and DVDs
Spinning class	Exercises using resistance bands and tubes	Meditation
Jumping rope, plyometrics, jumping boxes, active calisthenics like jumping jacks and "burpees," and similar heart-pumping gym activities	Strenuous yoga classes that focus on lifting your own body weight, like Ashtanga and power yoga	Deep breathing
Active yoga styles like vinyasa, flow yoga, or Bikram	Classes that use weights, like BodyPump	Stretching classes and DVDs

Many exercise programs cover all three types of exercise in one, like:

- Classes offered at fitness centers that incorporate cardio, strength, and stretching, or at least two of these (you can always take care of the missing element while you're at the gym). There are a lot of them out there.

- Barre/ballet classes that incorporate cardio, strength, and stretching.

- Thousands of exercise DVDs that include whole exercise systems you can do at home. Some will fit perfectly into your 30-minute lunch break, and some are as short as 10 minutes. There are also plenty of others that are less intense.

Creating Your 1:1:1 Exercise Plan

Now that you have a good idea which kinds of exercise fall into which category, it's time to make a plan. First, there are a few strategies to keep in mind, no matter how you construct your workout:

- Hydrate according to 1:1:1. Drink at least 8 ounces of water during the 30 minutes before your workout, at least 8 ounces after exercise (bring your water bottle and sip often), and at least 8 ounces during the 30 minutes after you exercise.

- Have a snack before exercise and a snack or meal after exercise. Never wait too long to eat after exercising. If you work out first thing in the morning, you still need a preworkout snack.

- Exercise at least three times a week, depending on which plan you choose.

- Always take at least 1 day off from exercise per week. Work out 6 days at most! Your body needs rest in order to recover and get stronger.

- If you're on 1:1:1 Accelerated, you want to accelerate your workout, too! Do one more workout a week than you're currently doing. For example, if you already work out 3 days a week, bump it up to 4. The only exception: If you already work out 6 days a week, keep your rest day. Instead, add an extra hour to your workouts in small chunks—divide 60 minutes by how many days you exercise, and add that time to each workout.

Personalizing 1:1:1

Now it's time to determine what kind of exercise plan you'll do. If you aren't exercising already, it's a good idea to start with short exercise sessions, light weights, and gentle stretches. Work up to longer sessions and higher intensity as you get more fit. If you're already exercising, jump in at a level at or slightly above where you are now, as you rebalance your workout.

I recommend approaching the construction of your 1:1:1 workout in one of three ways. Choose whichever one of the following three plans works best with your schedule, your preferences, and your life. Or switch back and forth from week to week, to keep things interesting. Nobody ever said you had to keep your routine the same every week!

The 20:20:20 Plan

On this plan, you'll balance your workout by piecing together all three elements yourself, just the way you might construct a meal or a snack. You'll exercise for an hour at a time at least 3 days per week, broken up as follows:

- 20 minutes of cardio, such as walking or running on the treadmill or elliptical trainer, walking or running outside, pedaling a real or stationary bicycle, or doing 20 minutes of an aerobics-style video at home.

- 20 minutes of resistance training, such as lifting weights, using weight machines at the gym, doing squats and pushups and other calisthenics that use your own body weight, or doing a resistance-training DVD at home. Don't forget to work your abs—include 20 to 50 crunches or other ab exercises.

- 20 minutes of stretching, at the end of your workout. This could include basic, gentle stretching of the muscles you've been working or some yoga poses. Your gym may have a class you can take, or you could use a DVD if you don't want to create your own routine.

People with gym memberships often prefer this plan because it's easy to go from cardio machine to weight machine to the mat for stretching. This is also a good plan for beginners, who may not want to do one thing for very long, to avoid injury. It's flexible and it doesn't feel overwhelming.

The 3-in-1 Plan

On this plan, you find a workout class or DVD that includes all three types of exercise in one workout. Do it three times a week at first. Work up to more if you enjoy it (but remember that you need at least one rest day). Some good examples might be:

- An aerobics class or workout DVD that starts and ends with stretching and includes floor exercises for muscle building after the cardio portion. Cross-fit, CardioPump, and Xtend Barre classes are good examples, but many regular, generic aerobics classes follow this format.

- A yoga class that includes vigorous movement for cardio, poses that lift body weight, and stretching. Some examples include hot yoga, vinyasa yoga, or Ashtanga yoga. (Classes differ by teacher and method, so try a few to be sure the class covers all your bases, or ask the studio which classes cover all three aspects.)

This is a good plan for people who want to get in and get out without thinking about it too much. It's one-stop shopping and it takes no planning. You just show up, do what the instructor (or the instructor in the DVD) tells you to do, then get on with your day. This is also a good plan for beginners who are still learning what kind of exercise they like and/or who want guidance to be sure they exercise safely. You can try a new class or a new DVD every week.

Food for **Thought**

Did you know that even if you get regular exercise, sitting for more than 4 hours a day in front of any screen increases your risk of cardiovascular disease by 125 percent? In fact, several studies have demonstrated that the longer you sit, the greater your risk of obesity, heart disease, and diabetes. Lack of exercise has also been linked to higher cancer risk and higher rates of depression. In other words, it's not just that exercise is good. It's that a lack of exercise is actively harmful to your health! So, about that walk you were going to take today . . . ?

The 3-or-6 Plan

On this plan, you choose to work out either 3 days per week (especially if you're just starting or restarting to exercise) or 6 days a week (if you're already exercising and want to ramp up your intensity). Then, on each of these 3 or 6 days, you perform 30 to 60 minutes of cardio, strength training, or stretching—one type of workout per day, per session. Pick the amount of time that works with your schedule and your fitness level. If 30 minutes feels like plenty, keep your workouts to 30 minutes until they feel too easy. If you're fit and you can squeeze it in, aim for an hour. As long as you keep your cardio, strength-training, and stretching sessions equal in length, you will stay in balance. Avoid overexercising, which could exhaust you, put your body in a state of stress, and increase your chance of injury.

Here are some ways the 3-or-6 Plan might work.

If you exercise 3 days per week:

- 30 minutes on the elliptical trainer on Monday, 30 minutes of weight training on Wednesday, and a 30-minute relaxing stretching class on Saturday

- 45 minutes of running on Tuesday, 45 minutes working with kettle-bells and free weights on Thursday, and a 45-minute yoga DVD at home on Saturday

- 1-hour Zumba class on Monday, 1-hour BodyPump class on Wednesday, and 1-hour yoga class on Friday

If you exercise 6 days per week:

- 30 minutes on the treadmill on Monday and Thursday, 30 minutes on the weight machines on Tuesday and Friday, 30 minutes of yoga on Wednesday and Saturday

- 45 minutes of brisk walking on Monday and Friday, a 45-minute weight workout with dumbbells at home on Tuesday and Thursday, and 45 minutes of yoga at home on Wednesday and Sunday

- Zumba class on Monday, Pilates class on Tuesday, Spin class on Wednesday, BodyPump class on Thursday, yoga class on Friday, meditation class on Sunday

The options really are endless. It's just like eating with 1:1:1. You get to pick the activities you love and piece them together to create a balanced, sensible, effective plan that will keep you in the best possible shape without overdoing it or underdoing it in any one area.

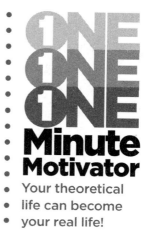

ONE ONE ONE Minute Motivator

Your theoretical life can become your real life!

The bottom line is that nobody can make you exercise, but if you want to do more than lose weight—if you want to look fit and toned and feel great, with increased confidence and energy—then you should add exercise to your life. Balance it with 1:1:1, and before long, it won't feel like a chore at all. You won't want to go through your week without it.

CHAPTER ELEVEN

The 1:1:1 Stress Reduction Plan

S*tress* may sound like a somewhat nebulous term, but technically, it's a very specific physical reaction to certain kinds of external situations. When you encounter something your brain perceives as threatening (a confrontation, a dangerous or scary situation, or a seemingly impossible task), it sends a message to your adrenal glands, which in turn pump out what are called stress hormones, like cortisol and adrenaline. This process launches you into "fight or flight" mode: Your heart and breathing rates increase, blood is shunted to your muscles, your blood sugar increases so you have more energy, and you become hyperalert—all physiological changes that prepare you to run away from or fight back against whatever's threatening you.

That's all good if you're being followed and you have to sprint to safety or use your best kickboxing moves to defend yourself. It also comes in handy if you're working to meet a tight deadline or have to give a speech in front of an audience—you'll be more alert, focused, animated. The trouble occurs when you're under pressure most of the time on most days—unfortunately, a situation too many people find themselves in. Your body is continually being bathed in stress hormones, and this has a negative impact on your health—increasing blood pressure and inflammation that leads to diseases like heart disease and diabetes, and increasing your weight.

Chronic stress messes with your willpower because it affects the way your prefrontal cortex processes information. This is the area of the brain that performs "executive functions" such as decision making, planning, making moral judgments, controlling behavior, problem solving, and goal setting. So proper prefrontal cortex function is crucial! When your ability to plan, set goals, or control behavior is compromised, you aren't going to be making great decisions about what to eat or when to exercise.

But beyond weakening your willpower, stress also sets off a chain reaction in your body that makes weight loss virtually impossible—*even if you eat right*. The stress hormones cortisol and adrenaline decrease the body's sensitivity to leptin, another hormone that signals your brain that you're full and tells you to stop eating. This means that when you're stressed out, you're much more likely to overeat because your body isn't sending you the normal "I'm full" cues.

That's not all, though. Stress hormones disrupt the normal blood sugar/insulin cycle, just when you need it to be working best because you're more likely to be overeating due to the dampened leptin effect. More glucose remains unprocessed in your blood, so what does your body do? It stores it for later in the form of fat. Once the body's glucose storage capacity has reached its limit, much of the excess ends up in abdominal fat cells, which have the bad habit of releasing more hormones that encourage more belly fat. It's a self-perpetuating stress cycle that makes slimming down especially challenging, especially when it comes to that muffin top.

Bummer, right?

Maybe you're not surprised. I bet you've found yourself reaching for comfort foods like macaroni and cheese, pizza, cookies, or ice cream after a bad day, and waking up with a poochy stomach. Or, like many of us, you've plowed through a bag of chips like a wood chipper chewing up branches when you were anxious or angry (people tend to turn to crunchy foods to soothe these emotions), then felt exhausted and grouchy (and guilty!). Certainly studies show that stress leads to overeating, which leads to weight gain. Harvard University researchers found that women in particular were more likely to gain weight when facing financial problems, difficult jobs, strained family relationships, or the feeling that they were limited by their circumstances. Weight-gain-related

1 1 1

Stress-Less Strategies

Feeling stressed? Here are some quick ways to feel better fast—all with zero calories!

- Go for a 15-minute walk.

- Stop what you're doing and listen to a song you love.

- Take a bath.

- Get a massage, pedicure, or facial.

- Turn off your smartphone and log out of your e-mail program for 1 hour.

- Hang out with your child for 20 minutes. Focus on nothing else. (If your child is a teenager, this may or may not work for stress relief!)

- Spend 15 minutes petting and playing with your dog or cat.

- Meditate or pray.

- Take 30 minutes and go read a magazine or a book chapter.

- Write in your journal about what's making you feel stressed (one study demonstrated that writing about your problems actually makes them feel less like problems).

stressors for men primarily centered on work, especially when men felt they had no authority to make decisions or ability to learn new skills on the job. Also, those already overweight were more likely to gain *more* weight under stress.

But you and I both know overeating isn't the answer. When you're stressed, your body needs balance—and the 1:1:1 plan—more than ever, but to make good decisions and maintain your portion control, the first order of business is to manage your stress.

You may not be able to do anything about your high-pressure job, your rocky relationship, your insecure financial situation, your unruly children (or parents!), your unpleasant living situation, or your general-ized anxiety that your life isn't what you want it to be right now. But you can put a damper on the stress these situations cause and control your weight in the process. How? Simple. All you have to do is de-stress according to 1:1:1.

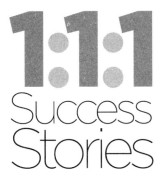

Name: **John Caruso**
Starting weight: **177 pounds**
Current weight: **160 pounds**
HEIGHT: **5'11"**

I used to be an emotional eater. I went for the sweets first and asked questions later. I exercised regularly, but always used my "active lifestyle" as an excuse to indulge. But afterward I would feel guilty and depressed. The 1:1:1 plan changed all that for me.

When I first met Rania, I had just been on a diet that left me emotionally drained and ready to give up on weight loss. Not only was I eating too few calories, but I wasn't getting enough nutrients and I was losing touch with what it meant to eat normally. I travel internationally a lot for work, so I needed a flexible approach to

The 1:1:1 of Stress Relief

Here's the thing about stress: People have all sorts of ways of coping with it, but the truth is that nothing works as well as a balanced approach to stress relief, one that employs the most effective methods in equal measure. Just as you should balance protein, carbs, and fat, you also need to balance your stress management techniques: contemplation, meditation, and respiration! To be more specific, you need to:

1. Contemplate what's causing your stress so you can start to change it, or at least change your attitude about it. In fact, feeling that you're in control often distinguishes good stress from bad stress.

2. Meditate, to foil the stress response at the source: in your brain. Your brain is what triggers the stress response, telling your adrenal glands to release stress hormones. Meditation trains your brain to respond

---

eating healthfully—a strategy I could use anywhere and everywhere. I wanted to lose weight and feel better, but I didn't think I would be able to find a plan that would fit my lifestyle and not leave me feeling deprived.

Rania's plan does what I need it to do. It's a realistic way of eating that I love. I couldn't believe I could eat whatever I wanted and still lose weight! With the 1:1:1 strategy, I finally understand how to balance what I eat, and when I do indulge in something sweet, I don't have to feel guilty about it because it's under control. Instead, I feel nourished, fueled, and satisfied. I've also found a balance between food and exercise. I have a sense of peace about my life that I never did before the 1:1:1 plan. I have lost 17 pounds and have maintained it for 2 years now. Plus, I was able to get the kind of definition in my abs that I was looking for. I'll never stop balancing my life with 1:1:1. For me, it's the ultimate formula.

more calmly and rationally to things that aren't really worth stressing about, so you can head off a stress response at the pass.

3. Breathe, which actually reverses the stress response in the body, signaling your brain, adrenal glands, muscles, and the rest of your body that there's actually no emergency. For example, let's say you're nervous about speaking in public. People in an emergency have quick, shallow breathing. People who are calm and relaxed breathe slowly and deeply. If you consciously breathe more deeply, your brain will realize that you aren't actually in danger and you'll feel calmer. Let's further examine these concepts.

Contemplation

Why are you stressed? What's really at the root of that anxiety? Why can't you relax? If you accept stress as your natural state and never look into it, it's not going to go away, and your muscles can't stay in that scrunched-up position forever without some cramping. Your organs can't function at peak capacity in emergency mode for years on end. If you don't get to the bottom of your stress, any stress-relieving technique will only deliver temporary relief. You need a fix.

My clients often complain to me that there's no way to "fix" the source of their stress. They can't quit their job, magically make their teenagers grow up and become responsible, or cause their spouses to stop leaving dirty laundry on the bathroom floor. True! Contemplating your stress isn't *necessarily* about fixing the cause. It's about understanding what the cause really is—which could lead to a solution, or at least to a realization that the source of stress really isn't as worthy of stress as you thought it was.

First, let's think about how you can fix a stressor. If you didn't even realize that you're stressed because your kitchen is always messy, then recognizing the effect of that messiness on you (not to mention how it stops you from cooking something healthy, which is why you're always ordering pizza) can be exactly the kind of motivation you need to develop a system to keep it cleaner. If you realize that cleaning the kitchen is all it takes to make you feel calmer, you might also realize it's not that hard.

Of course, when it comes to cleaning (and the stress that messes cause), getting help will make things easier. Sometimes, you have to get over that "I can do it all myself" mode that so many moms embrace—a source of stress in itself!—and be frank with your family or roommates. Tell them that you can't keep the kitchen clean alone, and you need some assistance. Delegate simple jobs at first. Whatever it takes. Walking into a clean, uncluttered kitchen in the morning can start your day out in a much nicer way. Aren't you feeling less stressed just *contemplating* that?

Maybe the cause of stress is a relationship, whether romantic or with a friend or family. You can't control how other people behave, but you can control how *you* behave—by doing something as simple as being less reactive, or by doing something life-changing, like ending the relationship. Contemplation gives you the opportunity to look more closely at your own role in any relationship conflicts. That other person may do something really aggravating, but do you respond in a way that escalates or diffuses the tension? Stress begins in your brain, not in the dirty laundry on the bathroom floor. It's just laundry. Stress comes out of your reaction to the laundry. If you decide to see it as proof of your partner's supreme incompetence or insistence on aggravating you, then you'll feel stressed. If you decide to see it as laundry on the floor, then you can either pick it up or ask your partner to pick it up without turning it into a stress-escalating argument. I'm not a psychologist, so I'm not going to get into detail about the many ways you can learn to reframe reactionary behavior. But I do counsel people enough to know that when you *react*

Food for **Thought**

Stress can deplete vitamin D stores by blocking your body's ability to efficiently absorb it. This vitamin (actually, it's a hormone) helps you absorb calcium, grow bone, prevent cancer, foil depression, lose extra weight, and keep your immune system functioning properly. So relax! And make sure you get enough daily D. A supplement and/ or 10 to 15 minutes of sun on your skin (without sunblock) should do the trick, or spend more time outside walking or gardening.

instead of *respond*, you're more likely to jack up your own stress level, as well as get into an argument. Contemplate that.

Meditation

People have a lot of preconceived notions about meditation, but it doesn't have to be "woo-woo," mystical, or even spiritual. The real benefit in meditation for stress relief is that it's basically a workout for your brain. You lift weights for your skeletal muscles, you do cardio for your heart muscle, and you meditate for your brain "muscle." Meditation is kind of like cross-training. You don't usually use your brain this way, so meditating gives your brain more range and flexibility. A study jointly conducted by Harvard University and the Massachusetts Institute of Technology found that subjects trained to meditate over an 8-week period had better control over the alpha rhythms in their brains. This control is related to concentration and the ability to minimize distractions, which means meditation can help you get better at focusing. Another study showed that people who meditated actually changed the structure of their brains—they had more gyrification, a folding of the tissues in the cerebral cortex linked to faster processing of information and better ability to make decisions, form memories, and pay attention. Meditation has been linked to increased "gray matter density in the brain stem," a structural change thought to relate to improved cognition, emotional responses, and even immune system responses, as well as better control over breathing and heart rate, which are directly linked to the stress response. A recent study also linked meditation to a better expression of the brain metabolites specifically related to anxiety and depression than in healthy people who didn't meditate, suggesting that meditation can keep those negative states under better control. I could go on and on, but you get the picture: Meditation helps you use your brain better.

On a practical level, meditation also gives your brain a break from constant obsessive thinking about every single thing. (We all do it.) By doing something your brain doesn't normally do, you get a rest from the things you *do* normally do. It's like you've been doing squats every day for a year. Now you finally spend a day doing biceps curls and chest presses.

Meditation can sound complicated, but it's not actually complicated at all. All you have to do is sit down, relax, and practice stilling your mind. Easier said than done, I know. Your brain isn't going to give up so easily. You've got a to-do list a mile long! I hear you! But give it a try because this is worthwhile. Here's a simple method that takes 5 minutes out of your life. Just 5 minutes! I just know you can spare that, for a good brain workout:

1. Sit down in a comfortable spot. You can sit on the floor like a Zen master if you want to, with or without a cushion, legs crossed, but it's not required. A chair is fine, too, if you need back support, as long as your feet are flat on the floor. (Lying down isn't a good position because it's too easy to fall asleep, but if you think you can stay awake, go for it.)

2. Set a timer for 5 minutes. Take a few deep breaths to calm yourself.

3. Rest your hands either on your knees or in your lap. Close your eyes.

4. Now, imagine a candle flame (or any small, simple object, if you don't like my candle idea). See it in your mind. Look at it. Focus on it. Don't think about anything else.

Food for **Thought**

In many people, the primary stress trigger is sleep deprivation. And people who get fewer than 7 hours of sleep every night tend to weigh more than those who get more sleep. Sleep seems to correlate with weight—the less people get, the more they weigh. One reason may be that people who don't get enough sleep have lower levels of leptin, a hormone that tells your brain when you're full. Without it, you may overeat, believing you aren't satisfied even though you've had enough food. Sounds like just one more good reason to catch some more ZZZs!

5. Of course, you'll think of everything else, but this is where the heavy lifting comes in. Every time you notice your mind has wandered, bring it back to that candle flame. Just gaze at it, in your mind's eye. Notice all the details—does it flicker or stay still? What color is it? What color is the candle? Keep bringing your mind back to the candle flame.

6. When the timer sounds, open your eyes, take a few refreshing breaths, and go on with your day.

This is a very simple meditation. As you get better at it, you can change the object of your focus and increase the amount of time you spend focusing. Boring? Maybe, but the benefits are amazing.

However, maybe focusing on an object isn't your style, just like step aerobics isn't your style. That's fine, too! Other ways to meditate are just as effective. Try one of these techniques, or switch them up and try a different one every time. Some people need to do a lot of different kinds of brain exercise to keep things interesting.

Food for **Thought**

Meditate, don't medicate! Meditation can improve your health in addition to calming your mind. A recent study by an insurance company looking at medical claims showed that people who meditated were hospitalized 30 percent fewer times for infectious diseases, 55 percent fewer times for benign and malignant tumors, and 87 percent fewer times for heart disease than people who didn't meditate. Also, meditation has been shown to lower blood pressure just as well as prescription drugs in those who have mild hypertension and to lower blood sugar levels in people with diabetes. Plus, meditation might even slow aging! In tests assessing chronological age versus "real age" based on biomarkers and habits, people who'd been meditating for 5 years or more averaged a real age 12 years younger than their chronological age. Sign me up!

- **Mantra meditation.** Instead of focusing on a mental picture, focus on a sound. This is called mantra meditation. The classic word is *Om*, and you can definitely use that, but you don't have to. Choose any simple word you like. A few suggestions: Peace, Love, Calm, God, Strong, Happy, or Clear. Slowly repeat the word, either out loud or in your mind. As soon as you notice your mind wandering, patiently bring it back to your mantra and keep repeating it until your time is up.

- **Visualization.** Instead of focusing on one object or sound, visualize a whole environment that relaxes you. It can be a place you've been to before, like your favorite beach or wilderness area, or it can be a place you invent. After closing your eyes, just start picturing it. Think of all the details. Imagine yourself walking there, or sitting there. Try to focus on as many details as you can. What do you see, hear, feel? Birds singing? The sound of breaking waves? Wind in the trees? A breeze on your face? The smell of flowers or wet sand? Totally immerse yourself in your visualized environment. If you start thinking about something else, bring your mind back to this "happy place" as soon as you notice you've strayed. Stay there, enjoying yourself, until your time is up.

- **Guided imagery.** There are a lot of great CDs, DVDs, and videos on the Internet that'll guide you through a meditation. Just sit down, relax, press Play, and let your mind do whatever the guide tells you to do. It might involve any one of the above techniques, or a combination of several.

- **Progressive muscle relaxation.** This is the one meditation you get to do lying down. Hooray! Starting at your feet, tense and then totally relax each body part, working your way up to your head. Give each part about 10 seconds: 5 seconds to tense the muscle, then 5 seconds to relax it. Flex and relax your feet, then your calves, thighs, abdomen, chest, hands, forearms, upper arms, shoulders, and finally, your face—scrunch it up and then relax it. Let yourself lie in this relaxed state for as long as you like.

- **Problem solving.** Your brain is a pretty amazing thing. It knows the answers to a lot of things you don't consciously know. If you can tap this knowledge, you can solve a lot of problems. This is a good meditation to do when something is really bothering you and you simply can't concentrate on anything else, let alone relax. All you have to do is sit quietly, breathe, close your eyes, then ask yourself the question: "What should I do about _____?" Then (here's the tricky part) don't answer your question. Your brain will want to leap to all kinds of answers, but those are just the surface-level answers you've already thought about. Instead, let your mind be quiet and just focus on the question. Wait. Wait. Wait for it. Once you've completely stopped trying to answer it on a conscious level, what often happens (somehow, miraculously) is that the answer simply floats up to the top of your consciousness like a bubble in a lake. Voila! Problem solved. It may not always work on the first try, but often works on the second or third. It's a great way to plumb your subconscious while also letting your mind work on a deeper level.

Food for **Thought**

I have an expression I use with my clients: M.E. time. It stands for motivation/energy time. I use this a lot when I work with moms, who tend to give away all their time and energy to their husbands and children and leave nothing for themselves. I believe in the power and importance of taking time for yourself to do whatever you want to do—not what you have to do, but simply what you enjoy. (Work doesn't count, even if you love your job.)

What about a date night or girls' night out, trip to the park with your kids, gym time, a good book, a walk, a bath. Or maybe waking up early to enjoy your coffee in silence, playing with your pets, planning your dream house, getting a massage or a pedicure, calling your sister, cooking or baking, or just hanging out with your partner or even by yourself, doing absolutely nothing at all.

This is recharge-your-batteries time, and it's important. You matter, not just to yourself, but to everyone who loves you and depends on you. They want you to be at your best, and this is what it takes.

Breathing

Deep breathing does something incredible—it actually reverses the stress response on a totally physical level. What happens when you panic? Your breath gets shallow and quick. Too much shallow, quick breathing can eventually lead to anxiety, or even a full-blown panic attack. Deep, slow breathing, however, has just the opposite effect. It signals your entire body that there's nothing wrong. That everything is fine. So fine, in fact, that you're just chilling out, so mellow that you're practically falling asleep.

This has profound effects on your physiology. Almost immediately (within a few breaths), your heart rate decreases, your blood pressure drops, and your muscles relax. Your adrenal glands can stop pumping out cortisol. You feel a sense of serene calm.

The goal is to take no more than 10 breaths in a minute. Here's how:

1. Use a watch or clock that keeps track of seconds. Sit comfortably, but make sure you sit up straight. You want to give your lungs plenty of room because you'll be breathing deeply.

2. Begin by breathing in for 3 seconds, then breathing out for 3 seconds. Do this for 1 minute. There you go—10 breaths. Easy, right?

3. Now make it more challenging. Breathe in for 4 seconds, then out for 4 seconds. Once this feels easy, try 5 seconds.

4. Eventually, see if you can work up to a 10-second inhalation and a 10-second exhalation. That's just three full breaths in a minute. Wow! You're looking so relaxed!

Another trick that yoga practitioners like to use is to make your inhalations and exhalations different lengths. You can put the stopwatch away for this one. Here's the general yoga rule of thumb.

• When your inhalation is longer, you'll feel energized. This is great for when you need to wake up and pay attention.

• When your exhalation is longer, you'll feel relaxed. This will help you unwind, calm down, or fall asleep.

Now try any of the following:

- Inhale to a slow count of five (about 5 seconds), then exhale normally. Repeat 10 times.

- Inhale normally, but exhale to a slow count of five (about 5 seconds). Repeat 10 times.

- Inhale to a slow count of three, then exhale forcefully, with a hissing sound, getting rid of all your air in one big push. Repeat 10 times. (This is very energizing!)

- Inhale quickly and fully, then exhale to a slow count of 10. (This is very good for calming down when you're anxious.)

Applying 1:1:1 to Your Stressful Life

Okay, so now you have all kinds of ideas for contemplation, meditation, and breathing, but how do you work them into your life in terms of 1:1:1? That's the easy part! You don't have to feel any pressure to sit and think about your problems for an hour every day, or meditate for 30 minutes every morning when you'd rather be sleeping, or deep-breathe every time you freak out. You *can* choose to do any of those things, but I find that managing stress in a balanced way is more realistic and sustainable in daily life. (How many days in a row are you actually going to sit down and meditate for 30 minutes?)

In the exercise chapter, I gave you several different ways to employ 1:1:1, so you could pick the one that fit best into your life. Same thing goes here. Choose any of the following scenarios. Pick the one that feels the most natural to you, or mix it up and try different ones until you fall into a rhythm that works for you.

The 5:5:5 Plan

Got 15 minutes? I bet you do. Take just 15 minutes out of your day. (First thing in the morning? Lunch hour? Just before bed?) Get your timer. Sit down.

- Spend 5 minutes contemplating any sources of stress in your day and how you responded to them.
- Spend 5 minutes meditating, using any technique you like.
- Spend 5 minutes breathing deeply, using any technique you like.

There you go—your 15 minutes is divided into three equal parts. It's 1:1:1, done and done.

The 3-in-1 Plan

Many guided meditations incorporate quiet time in which you can practice contemplation, meditation using guided imagery, and deep breathing. Find a recording you really like that gives you the opportunity to do all three, and knock it all out in a more structured manner. You might also find a good meditation class or yoga class that includes meditation. Typically these will include some time for guided meditation and deep breathing, as well as some quiet space for contemplation. If your yoga class has a long Shavasana at the end (the part where you lie there on your mat relaxing), you could even get all three in.

The 3-or-6 Plan

Maybe it stresses you out to think about doing multiple kinds of stress relief at one time. Enough already with the multitasking! Then you might prefer the 3-or-6 plan: Choose either 3 or 6 days a week for stress relief. (I prefer 6, but my life is stressful. Wait . . . yours is too, right?) Each day, choose one of the three stress-relief methods: contemplation, meditation, or breathing, and do it for a set number of minutes, depending on what

Start-Now Strategy

Meditation sound too overwhelming? Too time-consuming? Just sit down for 1 minute and breathe slowly, inhaling and exhaling to a count of five. Only 1 minute. I know you have 1 minute.

works for you. Maybe you'll do just 5 minutes each time. Or 10. Or maybe you're all about this whole stress-relieving concept and you'll do an hour. Hey, if you've got the time, go for it! The trick is to make sure you do each one in balance for the same number of minutes per week. Here are some ways this might work out.

- 5 minutes on Monday of contemplation, 5 minutes on Wednesday for meditation, and 5 minutes on Friday for breathing exercises

- 10 minutes on Monday and Friday for contemplation (a good way to start and end your workweek), 10 minutes on Tuesday and Saturday (your least stressful days?) for meditation, and 10 minutes each on Wednesday and Thursday for deep breathing (to get you through that stressful midweek period)

- 30 minutes on Tuesday for contemplation, 30 minutes on Thursday for meditation, 30 minutes on Sunday for breathing

I'm sure you can think of a hundred other combinations. Just pick what works, keep to 1:1:1, and you'll be calm, cool, and collected all week long.

The more you work with 1:1:1, the more you may find opportunities to balance every part of your life, and I believe that more balance always leads to less stress. Life should be beautiful, pleasurable, fun, and celebratory—at least some of the time. So enjoy your food (in balance), enjoy moving your body (in balance), enjoy your relaxation time (in balance), and most importantly, enjoy your life! The key is 1:1:1: Learn it, use it, live it, and you'll get healthier, slimmer, stronger, fitter, calmer, and more in control of everything about your life. Because that's the bottom line, isn't it? You want a better life than you have today. And you can get it! Just stick with 1:1:1, and you'll realize that you have won, won, won!

CHAPTER TWELVE
1:1:1 Recipes

love to cook and I love to eat good food, which is why I never recommend or eat diet-y food or serve it to my family. I believe that making healthy meals should never involve removing flavor. Don't replace sugar with stevia, or butter with applesauce, or meat with soy, unless you really prefer the taste. Eat the real stuff. As long as you moderate your portions, your body will stay in proportion! (Or resume its natural proportions.)

These are all dishes I make for my family at home. They are delicious, nutritious, and easy to prepare, but one thing they definitely are not is diet-y.

I've given you 30 entrées here—that's a month's worth of dinners and lunches to keep you happy—along with 15 breakfasts, 15 sides, and 15 snacks. I've indicated whether each dish is a complete 1:1:1 meal or snack on its own and, if not, I've suggested how to make it so. I've also given guidelines to make each dish fit into the 1:1:1 Accelerated plan.

· Feel free to make any of these recipes your own with appropriate like-for-like substitutions. For instance, replace beef with chicken, red bell peppers with onions, corn tortillas with flour tortillas, or whatever you prefer. As long as you keep the 1:1:1 ratio intact, the recipes will remain exactly what you need to stay on track.

You may notice that some of these recipes contain more than one source of protein, carbs, or fat. Don't be alarmed! And don't let worries about dissecting every element of a recipe keep you from cooking. Whatever the recipe you love, if you have one serving, and add any missing elements, you will stay in balance, even if the recipe for your Berry French Toast Bake has two carbs (bread and berries). Maybe you'll garnish your Berry French Toast with Greek yogurt (protein) and cinnamon almonds (fat). Even though this recipe is made with two different foods that fall into the carb category (bread and berries), you would still count it as your one carb for the meal. It's fine.

That being said, I don't want you to start having half of this and half of that when assembling your own meals—half a slice of bread, half a cup of potato salad, to cobble together one carb serving. This DIY approach makes it too easy to expand those half-servings into slightly bigger and bigger portions until you are eating too much again. Just pick your carb and go with it. However, for a recipe, it's done for you. If you eat one serving, then portion control is under control, so don't worry about it. It's either 1:1:1 (like a pasta salad with chicken and walnuts, no matter what other small amounts of other ingredients it contains), or it's missing something like protein or fat, and then you add the missing element.

So please start cooking! Don't be afraid. Whether the recipe is from this book or from your grandmother's recipe box or your favorite food blog, the point is that you made it yourself from fresh ingredients. Hooray for you! Have your serving, make sure it's balanced, add what's missing, and move on with your life. The 1:1:1 is easy—no need to make it complicated. Just use your common sense and let a food be what it is.

If you are still confused, see page 150 to refresh your memory about how to count mixed foods, or just follow these recipes and our suggestions for what to pair with them. You'll stay balanced, satisfied, and have a slimmer waistline, too! A reminder about dessert: I haven't included any dessert recipes here. I figure you know what you like and you know that on the 1:1:1 plan you can have dessert with lunch or dinner and count it as your carb (unless you are on 1:1:1 Accelerated; then eat dessert at lunch only).

Breakfasts

Start your day out right with any of these recipes. Of course, you'll probably have your favorites, and there's nothing wrong with rotating between a couple of breakfasts on most days. But I encourage you to try something new on days when you have a little more time and energy.

Summer Farmers' Market Frittata

Serves 6

I've categorized this as a breakfast, but this savory frittata is also perfectly delicious for lunch or dinner. Follow the recipe exactly, or substitute the seasonal veggies that look freshest. You can make this ahead of time and reheat it just before serving. A slice also makes a great breakfast to take to work; just warm it in your office's microwave oven.

1 tablespoon extra virgin olive oil
$\frac{1}{2}$ cup chopped onion
$\frac{1}{2}$ cup chopped asparagus
$\frac{1}{2}$ cup chopped zucchini
$\frac{1}{4}$ cup thinly sliced sun-dried tomatoes
Sea salt
Freshly ground black pepper
12 eggs, lightly beaten
$\frac{1}{2}$ cup crumbled goat cheese
2 tablespoons crumbled feta cheese
$\frac{1}{4}$ cup thinly sliced fresh basil

1. Preheat the oven to 350°F. In a large ovenproof skillet, heat the oil over medium-high heat. Add the onion and cook, stirring occasionally, until soft and translucent, about 10 minutes.

2. Add the asparagus, zucchini, and tomatoes and cook, stirring occasionally, until soft, about 10 minutes. Season to taste with the salt and pepper. Transfer the mixture to a plate and set aside.

3. Reduce the heat to medium-low. In the same skillet, add the eggs and cook until just set, about 4 minutes.

4. Spread the reserved vegetable mixture on top of the eggs. Transfer the skillet to the oven and bake until the eggs are set, about 8 minutes. Scatter the goat cheese and feta cheese over the frittata during the last 2 minutes of cooking. Remove the frittata from the oven, let it cool slightly, and cut it into wedges. Garnish with basil.

Make it 1:1:1: Add a carb, such as a piece of fruit or a slice of toast at breakfast or a side of roasted potatoes at dinner.

Almond-Berry Muesli

Serves 2

This breakfast, served hot or cold, is a welcome change from your regular bowl of cereal.

- 1 apple, peeled and finely chopped
- $\frac{1}{2}$ cup rolled oats
- $\frac{1}{4}$ cup fresh blueberries, raspberries, or sliced strawberries
- $\frac{1}{4}$ cup chopped almonds
- 1 tablespoon freshly squeezed lemon or orange juice
- $\frac{1}{2}$ teaspoon ground cinnamon
- $\frac{1}{4}$ teaspoon sea salt
- 1 cup low-fat or fat-free milk, divided

In a bowl, combine the apple, oats, berries, almonds, juice, cinnamon, salt, and $\frac{1}{2}$ cup of the milk. Serve immediately, with an additional $\frac{1}{2}$ cup of milk on the side.

A single serving of this recipe is a complete 1:1:1 meal.

Protein Waffles

Serves 2

Adding protein and fat turns frozen waffles into a healthy breakfast. Choose whole grain waffles, if you like them.

1 frozen waffle
1 cup plain nonfat Greek yogurt
2 tablespoon nut or seed butter
1 teaspoon ground cinnamon

Toast the waffles. Meanwhile, in a small bowl, combine the Greek yogurt and the nut or seed butter. Spread each waffle with the yogurt mixture and sprinkle the cinnamon on top.

A single serving of this recipe is a complete 1:1:1 meal.

Old-Fashioned Milk and Honey Oatmeal

Serves 2

Steel-cut oats give this comforting breakfast more staying power. Enjoy their chewier texture—a nice contrast with the creamy milk and sweet honey.

1 cup steel-cut oats
$1\frac{1}{2}$ cups water
1 cup low-fat or fat-free milk
1 tablespoon honey
$\frac{1}{2}$ teaspoon ground cinnamon
$\frac{1}{4}$ teaspoon sea salt
$\frac{1}{2}$ cup chopped walnuts

1. In a medium saucepan, combine the oats, water, and milk. Bring to a boil, then lower the heat and add the honey, cinnamon, and salt.

2. Simmer, uncovered, until thickened, about 20 minutes. If the oatmeal is too thick, add more water to reach your desired consistency. Divide the oatmeal between 2 bowls and top each serving with the walnuts.

A single serving of this recipe is a complete 1:1:1 meal.

Whole Grain Fruited Scones

Makes 12 scones

These scones taste like pastries but are lighter and more nutritious than the scones in your local coffeehouse.

1½ cups whole wheat flour
1½ cups whole wheat pastry flour
½ cup rolled oats
¼ cup raw sugar
¼ teaspoon baking soda
⅓ cup cold butter, cut into small pieces
1½ cups low-fat buttermilk
1 cup dried cherries or golden raisins

1. Preheat the oven to 375°F. Lightly grease a baking sheet.

2. In a large mixing bowl, combine the whole wheat flour, whole wheat pastry flour, oats, sugar, and baking soda. Stir well. Using a pastry blender, cut in the butter until the mixture resembles coarse bread crumbs. Add the buttermilk, stirring until just combined. Add the dried fruit and gently mix until combined.

3. Turn the dough onto a lightly floured surface and knead it 10 times. Gently shape the dough into a 9-inch circle. Place it on the baking sheet and cut it into 12 wedges.

4. Bake for 30 to 35 minutes, or until golden brown. Serve warm or cooled.

Make it 1:1:1: Add a pat of butter and a fat-free latte.

Egg Salad with Pita

Serves 1

This is a quick, easy, on-the-go breakfast. If you boiled a dozen eggs at the beginning of the week, you could have this most mornings.

1 hard-cooked egg, peeled
1 tablespoon extra virgin olive oil or mayonnaise
Salt

Freshly ground black pepper
Dash of cumin
1 mini whole wheat pita

In a small bowl, mash the eggs. Drizzle the olive oil over the mashed eggs. Add the salt, pepper, and cumin to taste. Toast your pita and stuff it with the egg salad, or spread the egg salad on top.

A single serving of this recipe is a complete 1:1:1 meal.

Breakfast Pizza

Serves 8

You might not have had pizza for breakfast since college, but this version is nutritionist approved. Kids love this breakfast, and you will, too.

1 prebaked whole wheat pizza crust
2 cups (8 ounces) shredded mozzarella cheese, divided
8 eggs
¼ cup water
Cooking spray
½ cup finely chopped onion
½ cup thinly sliced mushrooms
¼ cup chopped green bell pepper
¼ cup chopped red bell pepper
1 clove garlic, minced
1 teaspoon dried oregano

1. Preheat the oven to 400°F. Put the pizza crust on a baking sheet. Spread ¼ cup of the cheese evenly over the crust. Set aside.

2. In a medium bowl, whisk the eggs with a fork until well combined. Add the water and whisk again to lighten the mixture.

3. Coat a nonstick skillet with cooking spray and set it over medium-high heat. Add the egg mixture, onions, mushrooms, red and green peppers, and garlic. Scramble the eggs until cooked through but still moist, about 8 minutes.

4. Spoon the egg and vegetable mixture evenly over the pizza crust. Top with the remaining cheese. Sprinkle the dried oregano evenly over the top.

5. Bake for 20 minutes, or until the center is hot and the cheese is completely melted. Remove from the oven and cool for 5 minutes. Cut the pizza into 8 slices and serve.

A single serving of this recipe is a complete 1:1:1 meal.

Chia Seed Chocolate Pudding

Serves 1

Who says you can't have chocolate for breakfast? Not me, especially when it's in the super-nutrient-dense form of chia pudding. You can find chia seeds in the health food aisle of your grocery store. They are rich in omega-3 fatty acids, which are great for your heart. (They count as your fat.) This breakfast is extra easy because you whip it up the night before and it transforms into pudding while you sleep.

> 1 cup low-fat or fat-free milk
> 1 tablespoon chia seeds
> 1 tablespoon real maple syrup or honey
> 1½ teaspoons cocoa powder
> ¼ teaspoon ground cinnamon

In a small bowl, combine the milk, chia seeds, maple syrup or honey, cocoa powder, and cinnamon. Mix well. Cover and refrigerate overnight. In the morning, dig in with a spoon!

A single serving of this recipe is a complete 1:1:1 meal.

Chai-Spiced Pancakes

Serves 4 (makes about 8 6-inch pancakes)

Exotically flavored and full of nutrition from whole grain flour and ground flaxseed, these pancakes will win over the whole family.

> 1 cup fat-free milk
> ½ cup brewed black tea (like English Breakfast)

½ cup plain nonfat Greek yogurt
2 tablespoons real maple syrup
2 tablespoons canola oil
2 cups whole wheat pastry flour
¼ cup ground flaxseeds
2 teaspoons baking powder
1 teaspoon baking soda
1 teaspoon ground cinnamon
½ teaspoon ground ginger
¼ teaspoon ground cardamom
¼ teaspoon ground nutmeg
¼ teaspoon salt
⅛ teaspoon ground cloves
Cooking spray
6 teaspoons butter
6 tablespoons maple syrup or honey

1. Preheat the oven to 250°F. In a medium mixing bowl, whisk together the milk, tea, yogurt, maple syrup, and oil.

2. In a large mixing bowl, mix together the flour, flaxseeds, baking powder, baking soda, cinnamon, ginger, cardamom, nutmeg, salt, and cloves.

3. Add the wet mixture to the dry mixture and stir until well combined, with no dry pockets left.

4. Coat a skillet or griddle with cooking spray and place it over medium heat. For each pancake, ladle approximately ¼ cup of the batter onto the hot skillet to make a 6"-diameter pancake. Cook until the edges are set and bubbles form in the center, about 2 to 3 minutes. Flip and cook until the bottom is golden brown, about 2 to 3 minutes longer. (Keep cooked pancakes warm in the oven until ready to serve.) Serve hot, topped with a pat of butter and 2 tablespoons maple syrup or honey per serving.

Make it 1:1:1: Add a protein, such as nut butter, chicken or turkey sausage, or a glass of milk.

Mediterranean Omelet

Serves 1

This omelet will have you dreaming about breakfasting on a terrace in Italy overlooking the Mediterranean.

1 egg
1 tablespoon water
1/4 teaspoon salt
1 teaspoon extra virgin olive oil
1/2 cup chopped marinated artichoke hearts
1/4 cup finely chopped fresh tomatoes
1 ounce grated Asiago cheese or
1 tablespoon finely chopped high-quality green olives
  (preferably from Italy or Greece)
1/4 cup finely shredded fresh basil

1. Heat a nonstick skillet over medium-high heat. In a mixing bowl, whisk the eggs with a fork. Whisk in the water until combined. Add the salt.

2. Add the olive oil to the hot skillet, then pour in the eggs. Tilt the pan so the eggs cover the bottom. Gently coax the edges loose with a spatula, to keep the omelet from sticking. Cook for about 3 minutes.

3. As the omelet cooks, top it with the artichoke hearts, tomatoes, cheese, and olives. Cook until the eggs are set, another 3 to 4 minutes. Carefully fold the omelet in half and ease it onto a plate. Garnish with the shredded basil.

Make it 1:1:1: Add a carb, such as orange slices sprinkled with cinnamon.

Good Morning Casserole

Serves 6

Whip this up the night before. Then all you have to do in the morning is preheat the oven and bake it!

Cooking spray
$\frac{1}{2}$ cup chopped onions
2 cloves garlic, minced
$\frac{1}{2}$ cup sliced mushrooms
$\frac{1}{4}$ cup finely chopped green bell peppers
1 pound turkey sausage links, sliced
1 cup fat-free milk
6 large eggs
$\frac{1}{2}$ teaspoon dried basil
$\frac{1}{2}$ teaspoon dried rosemary
$\frac{1}{2}$ teaspoon salt
Freshly ground black pepper
6 slices whole grain bread, cut into $\frac{1}{2}$" cubes

1. Coat a 13" x 9" baking dish with cooking spray and set it aside.

2. Coat a large skillet with cooking spray and place it over medium-high heat. Cook the onions and garlic, stirring frequently, until browned, about 3 minutes. Add the mushrooms and bell pepper. When heated through, add the sausage slices. Cook, stirring frequently, until the sausage is cooked through, about 12 minutes. Remove from the heat and cool slightly.

3. In a large bowl, whisk together the milk, eggs, basil, rosemary, salt, and pepper. Add the sausage mixture and the bread, stirring to combine. Pour the mixture into the baking dish. Cover and refrigerate for at least 8 hours.

4. Preheat the oven to 350°F. Uncover the dish and let the casserole stand at room temperature for 15 minutes. Bake for 50 minutes, or until the eggs are set and the top is lightly browned. Let rest for 10 minutes prior to serving.

A single serving of this recipe is a complete 1:1:1 meal.

P.B. Smoothie

Serves 1

Feel free to alter this recipe by using other fruits, like pineapple and mango. PB stands for "perfectly balanced."

> **2 cups frozen strawberries**
> **$\frac{1}{2}$ cup coconut water**
> **$\frac{1}{2}$ cup plain nonfat Greek yogurt**
> **1 tablespoon ground flaxseeds**
> **1 cup ice**

In a blender, place the banana, strawberries, coconut water, yogurt, flaxseeds, and ice. Puree until smooth. Serve immediately.

A single serving of this recipe is a complete 1:1:1 meal.

Barley-Oat Hot Cereal

Serves 4

This comforting cereal is a nice change of pace if you're tired of regular oatmeal. The barley adds an interesting flavor, and steel-cut oats give it a chewy texture. (Together they equal one carb per serving.)

> **4 cups water**
> **$\frac{1}{2}$ cup steel-cut oats**
> **$\frac{1}{2}$ cup semi-pearled barley**
> **$\frac{1}{4}$ cup chopped walnuts**
> **1 teaspoon honey**
> **1 teaspoon salt**
> **$\frac{1}{4}$ teaspoon ground cinnamon**
> **$\frac{1}{4}$ teaspoon ground nutmeg**

In a medium saucepan, bring the water, oats, barley, walnuts, honey, salt, cinnamon, and nutmeg to a boil. Reduce the heat and simmer, stirring occasionally, until the grains are tender, about 25 minutes. Serve hot.

Make it 1:1:1: Add a protein, such as 3 ounces sausage links or 2 slices turkey bacon.

Poached Eggs with Pepper Sauce

Serves 2

This flavorful recipe is my take on *shakshuka*, a delicious Tunisian dish. *Shakshuka* means "a mixture" in Arabic slang and "all mixed up" in Hebrew. If you love huevos rancheros, you'll love this recipe.

1 tablespoon extra virgin olive oil

1 small onion, chopped

1 clove garlic, finely chopped

2 red bell peppers, seeded and cut into $\frac{1}{2}$"-wide strips

2$\frac{1}{2}$ teaspoons sea salt, divided

1 medium tomato, cored and grated

1 cup water

1 tablespoon harissa (Tunisian hot chili paste), plus additional, to taste

1 teaspoon apple cider vinegar

4 eggs

2 ounces shredded pepper-Jack cheese

1. In a medium skillet over medium heat, add the olive oil. When the oil is hot, add the onion and cook, stirring frequently, until soft, about 5 minutes. Add the garlic and stir for 1 minute. Add the bell peppers and $\frac{1}{2}$ teaspoon of the sea salt. Cook, stirring frequently, until the peppers are wilted, about 8 minutes. Add the tomato, water, and harissa. Reduce the heat to medium-low and cook, stirring often and adding additional water if the sauce reduces too much, until the peppers are soft. Add another $\frac{1}{2}$ teaspoon sea salt and additional harissa, if desired. Lower the heat and keep warm.

2. Fill a large pan with water and place it over medium heat. Add the vinegar and the remaining 1$\frac{1}{2}$ teaspoons sea salt.

3. When the water is simmering, one by one, crack each egg into a teacup and gently slide it into the water. Reduce the heat to low. Poach the eggs until the whites are firm and the yolks are just set, or about 4 minutes.

4. Evenly divide the bell pepper mixture between 2 bowls and place 2 eggs on top of each. Garnish each serving with 1 ounce of cheese.

Make it 1:1:1: Serve with toast or toasted corn tortilla.

Mixed Berry French Toast Bake

Serves 12

This easy riff on French toast is perfect for a Sunday brunch. Although it includes eggs and fruit, this is a French toast dish, so it counts as a carb. The almond garnish counts as a fat.

Cooking spray
3 tablespoons butter, softened
1 baguette, cut into 24 slices
2 cups fresh berries, any type or a mixture
2¾ cups fat-free milk
2 tablespoons brown sugar
1 teaspoon almond extract
6 eggs
¼ cup slivered almonds

1. Coat an 11″ x 7″ baking dish with cooking spray. Butter one side of each baguette slice.

2. Place 12 of the baguette slices, buttered side down, in a single layer in the dish (it's alright if they overlap a little).

3. Sprinkle the berries over the bread in an even layer. Top with the remaining 12 bread slices, buttered side up.

4. In a bowl, whisk together the milk, sugar, almond extract, and eggs. Pour the mixture evenly over the baguette and berry mixture. Cover the baking dish and refrigerate for at least 8 hours.

5. When ready to bake, preheat the oven to 350°F. Sprinkle the casserole with the almonds. (This dish can go straight from fridge to oven.)

6. Bake for 45 minutes, or until the top is golden. Let rest for 5 minutes prior to serving.

Make it 1:1:1: Serve with a protein, such as turkey sausage patties.

Entrées

Have these for lunch or dinner, depending on your preference. I know you'll enjoy trying out some new flavors, as well as finding more balanced ways to cook familiar favorites. Happy cooking!

Greek Pasta Salad with White Beans

Serves 4

This recipe is a favorite with my clients. It's quick to prepare, filling, and satisfying because it has some exotic flavors but it still feels like comfort food.

10 ounces penne pasta
2 cans (15 ounces each) cannellini beans, rinsed and drained
2 tablespoons extra virgin olive oil, divided
1 clove garlic, minced
1 tablespoon fresh mint, chopped
1 teaspoon dried oregano, crushed
½ teaspoon sea salt
¼ cup freshly squeezed lemon juice
2½ cups baby spinach leaves
2 cups cherry tomatoes, halved
½ cup pitted kalamata olives or ½ cup crumbled feta cheese
Freshly ground black pepper

1. In a large pot of boiling salted water, cook the pasta according to package directions until al dente.

2. Meanwhile, in a small nonstick saucepan over medium heat, place the beans, 1 tablespoon of the olive oil, the garlic, mint, oregano, and salt. Cook, stirring occasionally, until heated through, about 5 minutes. Keep warm.

3. In a small bowl, whisk together the remaining 1 tablespoon of olive oil and the lemon juice to make a dressing.

4. Transfer the cooked pasta to a serving bowl. Top it with the beans, spinach, tomatoes, and olives (if using). Add the dressing and pepper to taste. Toss gently to combine. Sprinkle with the feta (if using) and serve.

A single serving of this recipe is a complete 1:1:1 meal.

1:1:1 Accelerated option: For dinner, skip the pasta—the beans serve as your carb and your protein. Serve over mixed greens. This is now a white bean salad!

Persian Chicken Stew

Serves 4

This delicious chicken stew tastes like it's hard to make, but it's actually quick and easy.

1 cup halved cherry tomatoes
2 bell peppers, cored, seeded, and cut into strips
1 cup coarsely chopped onions, divided
2 tablespoons extra virgin olive oil, divided
2 teaspoons sea salt
1 teaspoon ground cinnamon
1 teaspoon ground turmeric
1 teaspoon garlic powder
1 teaspoon brown sugar
1 teaspoon paprika
4 pieces bone-in chicken (such as 2 breasts and 2 thighs)
2 cloves garlic, minced
2 tablespoons tomato paste
$\frac{1}{2}$ cup hot water
Juice from 2 limes

1. Preheat the oven to 375°F.

2. In a 13" x 9" baking dish, place the tomatoes, bell peppers, and $\frac{1}{2}$ cup of the onions and drizzle with 1 tablespoon of the olive oil. Sprinkle the salt over the vegetables.

3. In a small bowl, combine the cinnamon, turmeric, garlic powder, brown sugar, and paprika.

4. Coat the chicken in the spice mixture. In a large skillet over medium heat, heat the remaining 1 tablespoon of oil. Cook the remaining ½ cup onion and the garlic, stirring frequently, until soft, about 10 minutes. Add the chicken and cook until browned on one side, about 4 minutes. Flip the chicken and cook until the other side is browned, about 4 more minutes. Place the chicken in the dish with the vegetables.

5. In a bowl, whisk the tomato paste, water, and lime juice until smooth. Pour over the chicken and vegetables. Bake for 40 minutes, or until a thermometer inserted in the thickest portion of the chicken registers 170°F and the juices run clear. Serve hot.

Make this a 1:1:1 meal: Add a carb. Serve over farro or with whole wheat lavash.

1:1:1 Accelerated option: For dinner, serve it over raw spinach or kale instead of adding a starchy carb.

Fava, Feta, and Flavor

Serves 4

This vegetarian dish is packed with protein, fiber, and, most of all, *flavor!* You can find sumac at Middle Eastern grocery stores, or you can substitute lemon pepper.

Cooking spray
1 eggplant, cut lengthwise into ¼-inch-thick slices
3 cloves garlic, minced
1 teaspoon dried oregano
Salt
Freshly ground black pepper
1 can (15 ounces) fava beans, rinsed and drained
5 cups mixed greens or spring greens
3 tablespoons sumac
1 tablespoon freshly squeezed lemon juice
1 tablespoon extra virgin olive oil
4 tablespoons crumbled feta cheese

1. Lightly spray a baking sheet with cooking spray. Preheat the oven to 425°F.

2. On the baking sheet, arrange the eggplant slices in a single layer. Sprinkle with the garlic, oregano, salt, and pepper. Bake the eggplant for 25 minutes, or until it begins to brown.

3. When the eggplant slices are cool enough to handle, cut them into bite-sized pieces. In a medium bowl, toss them with the fava beans.

4. Place the mixed greens in a large bowl. In a small bowl, whisk the sumac, lemon juice, olive oil, and salt and pepper to taste. Toss the greens with the dressing.

5. Divide the mixed greens among 4 bowls and top with the eggplant mixture. Sprinkle each serving with 1 tablespoon of the feta cheese.

Make it a 1:1:1 meal: Add a carb, such as half a whole wheat pita or a piece of whole wheat flatbread.

1:1:1 Accelerated option: No changes necessary.

Kale Taco Salad

Serves 2

This delicious salad is more nutritious than the typical taco salad, which is often made with iceberg lettuce, and the absence of a fried tortilla bowl makes it a slimmed-down choice (although you could choose a taco bowl as your carb).

10 ounces 85% lean ground beef
1 packet taco seasoning
¼ cup water
4 cups shredded kale
2 tablespoons tahini
1 tablespoon freshly squeezed lemon juice
2 tablespoons fresh salsa
Sea salt

1. In a large nonstick skillet over medium heat, place the ground beef. Sprinkle it with the taco seasoning and water. Cook, breaking the meat into smaller pieces with a stiff spatula, until browned, about 8 minutes.

2. Divide the kale between 2 bowls and top each with half of the beef mixture.

3. Whisk together the tahini and lemon juice until the tahini dissolves. Make sure that it's more liquid than pastelike in consistency. If it's too thick, whisk in a splash of water. Drizzle the dressing over the beef and kale.

4. Top each salad with a tablespoon of fresh salsa and sprinkle with salt to taste.

Make it 1:1:1: Add a carb, such as an ounce of tortilla chips or some baked pita wedges.

1:1:1 Accelerated option: No changes necessary.

Mediterranean Quinoa Bowl

Serves 1

This vegetarian meal is a good way to use up leftover quinoa. Tomatoes, fennel, broccolini, and arugula add Mediterranean flair in addition to nutrients such as vitamin A and lycopene.

$\frac{1}{2}$ cup broccolini
2 tablespoons dry quinoa
1 tablespoon extra virgin olive oil
$\frac{1}{2}$ cup halved cherry tomatoes
$\frac{1}{4}$ cup fresh, sliced fennel
1 clove garlic, chopped
$\frac{1}{2}$ teaspoon dried oregano
$\frac{1}{2}$ teaspoon dried basil
$\frac{1}{2}$ teaspoon salt
$\frac{1}{4}$ teaspoon freshly ground black pepper
1 cup chopped arugula
2 ounces feta cheese
$\frac{1}{4}$ cup pitted and chopped green olives
3 tablespoons chopped flat-leaf parsley

1. Bring a small saucepan of water to a boil and cook the broccolini until bright green, about 3 minutes. Cool, then tear into pieces.

Meanwhile, in a separate small pan, cook the quinoa according to package directions (or use ¹⁄₂ cup leftover cooked quinoa).

2. In a medium-sized pan over medium heat, heat the oil. Cook the tomatoes, broccolini, and fennel until tender, about 4 minutes. Add the garlic, oregano, basil, salt, and pepper and stir to incorporate. Remove from the heat.

3. In a serving bowl, layer the arugula, quinoa, vegetable and egg mixture, feta cheese, olives, and parsley. Serve warm.

A single serving of this recipe is a complete 1:1:1 meal.

1:1:1 Accelerated option: Enjoy as is for lunch only.

Thai-Inspired Fish en Papillote

Serves 4

Fish en Papillote is a French dish that translates, literally, as "fish in parchment." Cilantro, basil, ginger, soy sauce, and coconut milk move this dish east for a Thai flair. Mushrooms add vitamin D, while the brown rice adds filling fiber.

1 can (15 ounces) coconut milk
1 tablespoon soy sauce
1 tablespoon fish sauce
1 tablespoon freshly squeezed lime juice
2 teaspoons Thai green curry paste
1 cup brown or white rice
4 halibut, cod, or other white fish fillets
1 cup sugar snap peas
4 ounces button mushrooms, thinly sliced
4 scallions, thinly sliced
1 tablespoon grated fresh ginger
¹⁄₄ cup chopped fresh cilantro
¹⁄₄ cup chopped fresh basil
Salt
Freshly ground black pepper

1. Preheat the oven to 350°F. Whisk together the coconut milk, soy sauce, fish sauce, lime juice, and curry paste. Meanwhile, cook the rice according to package directions.

2. Cut out 4 heart-shaped pieces of parchment paper, each about 12″ wide. Put 1 fish fillet on each piece of parchment. Top each fillet evenly with the sugar snap peas, mushrooms, scallions, and ginger. Drizzle with the coconut curry sauce.

3. Fold over one side of each parchment paper, making a half-heart shape. Fold sharp creases all around each packet until it's completely sealed.

4. Bake for 15 minutes. Remove from the oven, cut the packets in half vertically, and peel apart the two sides. Garnish with the cilantro, basil, and salt and pepper to taste. Serve over the rice.

A single serving of this recipe is a complete 1:1:1 meal.

1:1:1 Accelerated option: **At dinner, serve this over shredded cabbage or salad greens instead of rice.**

ABC Tacos

Serves 6

The ABCs are avocado, black beans, and cilantro—a combo that will satisfy vegetarians and meat eaters alike! With the creamy avocado as your fat, you won't miss the cheese or sour cream.

Cooking spray
1$\frac{3}{4}$ cans (15 ounces) black beans, rinsed and drained
$\frac{1}{4}$ cup water
2 avocados, peeled, pitted, and finely chopped
1 cup halved cherry tomatoes
$\frac{1}{4}$ cup finely chopped scallions
$\frac{1}{4}$ teaspoon salt
6 corn or whole wheat tortillas
1 bunch fresh cilantro leaves, finely chopped
1 small lime, cut into 6 wedges

1. Preheat the oven to 325°F. Spray a nonstick skillet with cooking spray and cook the beans in the water over low heat until heated through.

2. In a medium bowl, mix the avocados, tomatoes, and scallions. Season with the salt.

3. On a large baking sheet, arrange the tortillas in a single layer. Bake for 5 minutes, or until heated through.

4. Remove the tortillas from the oven. Place $1/2$ cup of beans on each and top with the avocado mixture. Garnish each with cilantro and serve with a lime wedge. Serve hot.

A single serving of this recipe is a complete 1:1:1 meal.

1:1:1 Accelerated option: **Omit the tortillas and serve this over salad greens if having for dinner.**

Butternut Squash Curry

Serves 4

This flavorful dish is easy to make and you can use either chickpeas or chicken for your protein, depending on whether you want it to be vegan or not.

8 ounces cubed butternut squash
$1/2$ cup low-sodium chicken or vegetable broth
Cooking spray
$1/2$ cup chopped onion
4 scallions, white and green parts, chopped
$1/4$ cup slivered almonds
1 can (15 ounces) chickpeas, rinsed and drained, or 5 ounces cubed cooked chicken
$3/4$ cup Thai yellow curry sauce
$1/2$ cup cubed pineapple
$1/2$ yellow bell pepper, sliced
2 tablespoons golden raisins

1. In a large saucepan over medium heat, place the squash, the broth, and enough water to just cover the squash. Cook until the squash is soft, or about 15 minutes. Drain and set aside.

2. Spray a nonstick skillet with cooking spray. Add the onions, scallions, and slivered almonds and cook, stirring frequently, until the onions are soft, about 6 minutes.

3. Add the squash, chickpeas or chicken, curry sauce, pineapple, bell pepper, and raisins. Stir, and simmer until heated through, about 8 minutes.

Make it 1:1:1: **Serve with a carb, such as 1 cup couscous or a piece of naan per person.**

1:1:1 Accelerated option: **For dinner, serve with steamed vegetables or a salad or just enjoy a bowl topped with hot sauce.**

Black Bean Quinoa Salad

Serves 6

This is a heart-healthy, high-fiber, vegetarian, and gluten-free dish that's big on taste. It keeps well in the refrigerator for a few days. Freshen it up with lemon juice each time you are ready to serve it.

3/4 cup quinoa
2 cans (15 ounces each) black beans or chickpeas, rinsed and
  drained
Juice of 1 lemon
1/4 cup extra virgin olive oil
1/2 cup halved grape tomatoes
1/2 cup finely chopped red bell pepper
1/4 cup chopped scallions
Sea salt
Freshly ground black pepper

1. Cook the quinoa according to package directions.

2. In a large bowl, combine the cooked quinoa and the black beans or chickpeas. Drizzle with the lemon juice and olive oil. Toss to coat.

3. Add the tomatoes, bell pepper, and scallions, then season to taste with salt and pepper. Serve warm or cold.

A single serving of this recipe is a complete 1:1:1 meal.

1:1:1 Accelerated option: **Eliminate the quinoa and enjoy for dinner as a black bean salad.**

Lentil-Vegetable Loaf

Serves 6

My family loves this comforting, slimmed-down, vegetarian version of meat loaf.

1½ cups dried lentils
Cooking spray
¼ cup brown rice
1 cup chopped fresh mushrooms
¾ cup chopped onion
½ cup shredded carrot
½ cup chopped red bell pepper
½ cup wheat germ
¾ cup bread crumbs
½ cup raw, shelled, unsalted sunflower seeds
1 can (6.5 ounces) tomato sauce
1 egg, beaten
1 tablespoon extra virgin olive oil
2 teaspoons dried thyme
Pinch of ground red pepper
Sea salt

1. In a medium saucepan, place the lentils and enough water to cover them by 1". Bring to a boil and cook until tender, about 45 minutes. Check occasionally and add more water if needed. Drain and set aside to cool.

2. Preheat the oven to 375°F and spray an 8" x 4" loaf pan with cooking spray. In a medium pan, cook the rice according to package directions. In the bowl of a food processor, combine the mushrooms, onion, carrot, bell pepper, and wheat germ. Pulse until finely chopped. Transfer to a bowl and set aside.

3. Put the lentils in the food processor and process them into a paste.

4. Add the lentil paste to the bowl of chopped vegetables and then mix in the bread crumbs, rice, and sunflower seeds. Stir to combine.

5. Add the tomato sauce, egg, and oil. Stir to combine.

6. Season the mixture with the thyme, ground red pepper, and salt to taste. Stir to combine. Spoon it into the prepared loaf pan.

7. Bake for 45 minutes, or until heated through and browned on the top. Cool slightly before slicing and serving.

A single serving of this recipe is a complete 1:1:1 meal.

1:1:1 Accelerated option: **Reserve this meal for lunch rather than dinner.**

Couscous- and Chickpea–Stuffed Peppers

Serves 4

You can replace the chickpeas—your protein in this 1:1:1 meal—with ground turkey, lamb, or beef, if you prefer.

Cooking spray
4 large green bell peppers
1 tablespoon extra virgin olive oil
1 can (15 ounces) chickpeas, rinsed and drained
2 cups chopped onion, divided
1 green bell pepper, chopped
6 cloves garlic, minced
1 jar (16 ounces) chunky tomato sauce
1½ cups couscous
2 cups (8 ounces) shredded Monterey Jack or other white cheese
½ cup salsa

1. Preheat the oven to 375°F. Spray a 13" x 9" baking dish with cooking spray.

2. Cut the peppers in half vertically and remove their stems and seeds. Place them in the baking dish, cut side up.

3. In a large skillet over medium heat, cook the olive oil and chickpeas, stirring frequently, until heated through, about 5 minutes. Add

1½ cups of the chopped onion, the bell pepper, and the garlic. Reduce the heat to low, add the tomato sauce, and let simmer while preparing the couscous.

4. Prepare the couscous according to package directions, adding the remaining ½ cup of chopped onion to the water before adding the couscous. When the couscous is cooked, combine it with the chickpea mixture.

5. Fill the bell pepper halves with the chickpea mixture and top them with the cheese. Bake for 20 minutes or until the cheese is bubbly and slightly brown on top.

6. Top each pepper half with 1 tablespoon of salsa and serve.

A single serving of this recipe is a complete 1:1:1 meal.

1:1:1 Accelerated option: **Reserve this meal for lunch.**

Middle Eastern Lamb and Okra Stew

Serves 6

Stuck in a rut? Change things up with this delicious, exotic stew. It uses lamb and okra, two foods not as commonly consumed in the United States as beef, carrots, and onions. Variety is the spice of life!

2 tablespoons coconut, extra virgin olive, or canola oil, divided
½ teaspoon butter
2 pounds cubed lamb stew meat
4 cups water
1½ tablespoons tomato paste
1 can (16 ounces) diced tomatoes, drained
Sea salt
Freshly ground black pepper
1 teaspoon garlic powder
1 cube beef bouillon
2 pounds fresh small-to-medium okra
Fresh cilantro
3 tablespoons toasted slivered almonds

1. In a large sauté pan over medium heat, heat 1 tablespoon of the oil and the butter. Add the lamb and cook, turning occasionally, until all sides of the lamb are browned, about 7 minutes.

2. In a large saucepan, bring the water to a boil. Dissolve the tomato paste in the water, then add the diced tomatoes.

3. Add the salt, pepper, and garlic powder. Add the beef bouillon cube and stir to dissolve.

4. Add the cooked lamb to the tomato sauce mixture and bring to a boil. Lower the heat, cover, and simmer for 40 to 50 minutes.

5. While the stew is cooking, cut the stems off the okra. In a large skillet over medium heat, heat the remaining 1 tablespoon oil. Cook the okra, stirring frequently, until the ridges are brown, about 10 minutes. Season to taste with additional black pepper and salt.

6. Add the sautéed okra to the stew and mix gently. Simmer for an additional 15 minutes. Garnish with fresh cilantro and slivered almonds and serve.

Make it 1:1:1: Add a carb and a fat. Serve over 1 cup of basmati rice.

1:1:1 Accelerated option: No changes necessary.

Tahini Twister

Serves 1

Make extra veggies the night before and use the leftovers as your filling. You can add baby spinach or baby kale as well.

1 ounce feta cheese
1 tablespoon chopped fresh flat-leaf parsley or cilantro, or a combination of the two
1 whole wheat tortilla
1 tablespoon tahini
1 cup raw or cooked sliced vegetables, such as carrots, bell peppers, and cabbage

1. In a medium bowl, mix the feta with the parsley and cilantro.

2. Spread the tortilla with the tahini.

3. Add the vegetables and sprinkle with the feta cheese mixture. Wrap the tortilla around the filling, and serve.

A single serving of this recipe is a complete 1:1:1 meal.

1:1:1 Accelerated option: Reserve this for lunch.

Poached Fish or White Beans with Tomatoes and Kale

Serves 4

Cooking the kale in this tomato mixture keeps all of its nutrients intact. The white bean option is great for vegetarians or anyone.

2 tablespoons extra virgin olive oil
$\frac{1}{2}$ yellow onion, sliced
3 cloves garlic, minced
1 can (28 ounces) diced tomatoes
1 can (15 ounces) white beans, drained and rinsed
1 bunch kale (any type), stems removed, leaves chopped
$\frac{1}{3}$ cup vegetable or seafood broth
4 cod, halibut, or other white fish fillets (or 1 can white beans)
Sea salt
Freshly ground black pepper
$\frac{1}{2}$ cup chopped fresh basil

1. In a large skillet over medium-high heat, heat half the oil. Add the onion and cook, stirring frequently, until soft, about 4 minutes. Stir in the garlic and tomatoes. Cook, stirring occasionally, for 5 minutes.

2. Lower the heat to medium. Add the beans (if using), kale, and broth. Bring to a simmer and cook until the kale is completely wilted, about 20 minutes.

3. Reduce the heat to low. Place the fish fillets (if using) on top of the tomato mixture and cover the pan. Poach until the fish is cooked through and opaque, about 10 minutes. Season with the salt and pepper, garnish with the basil and remaining olive oil, and serve.

Serve with a cup of risotto to make this a complete 1:1:1 meal.

1:1:1 Accelerated option: **No changes necessary.**

Thai Chicken Noodle Dinner

Serves 4

In this pad-Thai-like dish, I use shredded carrots to replace half of the noodles, which bumps up the fiber. Enjoy with chopsticks—you just might eat slower!

4 cups water
1 package (8 ounces) rice noodles
⅓ cup creamy peanut butter
1 tablespoon freshly squeezed lime juice
1 tablespoon soy sauce
Cooking spray
2 cups cubed chicken breast
1 cup shredded carrots
2 tablespoons chopped fresh cilantro
Lime wedges

1. In a 3-quart saucepan, bring the water to a boil. Remove from the heat and add the noodles. (Make sure the noodles are covered completely with water. Push them under with the back of a spoon, if necessary.) Soak the noodles until they are soft but firm, or up to 5 minutes. Drain the noodles and rinse them with cold water. Set aside.

2. In a medium bowl, whisk together the peanut butter, lime juice, and soy sauce until smooth. Set aside.

3. Spray a large skillet with cooking spray and heat it over medium-high heat. Cook the chicken, stirring frequently, until the center is no longer pink, about 5 minutes. Add the peanut butter sauce and bring to a boil, stirring frequently. Stir in the noodles and carrots until thoroughly mixed. Cook, tossing with 2 wooden spoons or tongs, until thoroughly heated and the noodles are tender, about 3 minutes.

4. Sprinkle with cilantro. Serve with the lime wedges.

A single serving of this recipe is a complete 1:1:1 meal.

1:1:1 Accelerated option: For dinner, omit the rice noodles and serve this over shredded cabbage.

Eggplant Casserole

Serves 8

This casserole is my 1:1:1 take on the traditional Lebanese dishes of *makdous* (stuffed eggplant) and *fatet batinjan,* which contains egg-plant, yogurt, and fried bread. I use beef here, but you could also use lamb or veal. If you have leftovers, they'll reheat beautifully. Just pop them in the oven for 10 minutes and serve with fresh yogurt.

3 large eggplants

Sea salt

4 tablespoons extra virgin olive oil, divided

Freshly ground black pepper

1½ teaspoons garlic powder, divided

3 large pitas

1 teaspoon butter

1 pound beef stew meat

4–5 cups water

12 ounces tomato paste

3 cups plain nonfat Greek yogurt

¼ cup freshly squeezed lemon juice

2 tablespoons tahini

½ cup toasted pine nuts

½ cup chopped flat-leaf parsley

1. Preheat the oven to 400°F. Slice the eggplants into rounds. (Don't peel them, as the skin will help hold them together as they cook.) Sprinkle the eggplant rounds with salt and put them on a paper towel to absorb some of their moisture.

2. Brush the bottom of a 13″ x 9″ baking dish with 1 tablespoon of the olive oil and place the eggplant rounds in it.

3. Brush the tops of the eggplant rounds with 1 tablespoon of olive oil and sprinkle with salt, pepper, and garlic powder to taste. Bake for 40 minutes, or until golden. Remove from the oven and set aside.

4. While the eggplant is baking, cut the pitas into triangles and place in a bowl. Drizzle with 1 tablespoon of olive oil, salt, and ½ teaspoon garlic powder. Toss until each piece is coated. Place on a baking sheet and bake for 7 minutes, or until golden brown and crunchy. (Alternatively, you can make the pita chips the day before you bake the eggplant.)

5. In a medium skillet over medium heat, heat the remaining tablespoon of olive oil and the butter. Cook the beef until golden brown, or about 15 minutes.

6. In a large pot, bring the water to a boil. Add the tomato paste and stir to dissolve. Add the beef and lower the heat to low. Simmer until the beef is tender, about 45 minutes. Taste the sauce and season with salt and pepper, as needed.

7. While the beef is cooking, make the topping: In a small bowl, stir together the yogurt, lemon juice, and tahini with the remaining garlic powder. Season to taste with salt and set aside.

8. Take the beef off the heat and add the cooked eggplant to the pot. Cover the pot, letting the heat of the stew warm the eggplant.

9. Wash the baking pan you used for the eggplant, then spread the baked pita pieces in it. Pour the eggplant and beef stew over them. Top the casserole with the yogurt mixture. Garnish with the pine nuts and parsley and serve.

A single serving of this recipe is a complete 1:1:1 meal.

1:1:1 Accelerated option: **Make this casserole without the pita chips if you plan to have it for dinner.**

Kibbeh Bil Sanieh

This is a delicious Mediterranean dish, and there are as many ways to prepare it as there are cooks! Depending on how it's prepared, kibbeh can be served like meatballs or egg-shaped patties. This meat pie version is much easier!

> 2 cups very fine bulgur
> Cooking spray
> 3½ pounds 90% lean ground beef, divided
> 1 teaspoon ground allspice
> ¼ teaspoon ground cinnamon
> Freshly ground black pepper (liberal black pepper is great in this recipe!)
> Salt
> 1 large onion, chopped
> ½ cup toasted pine nuts
> 1 tablespoon extra virgin olive oil
> 8 lemon wedges
> 8 tablespoons plain nonfat Greek yogurt
> Flat-leaf parsley sprigs, for garnish

1. In a large bowl, soak the bulgur in just enough warm water to cover for 25 minutes (or overnight). The bulgur should absorb all the water and will almost double in size. Drain, and squeeze out any excess moisture.

2. Preheat the oven to 350°F and spray a 13″ x 9″ baking dish with cooking spray.

3. In a large bowl, mix the soaked bulgur and 1½ pounds of the ground beef. Season with the allspice, cinnamon, black pepper, and salt. Spread half of the mixture evenly in the prepared baking dish and set aside.

4. In a skillet over medium heat, cook the remaining 2 pounds of ground beef (not mixed with bulgar), breaking up the pieces with a spatula, until browned, about 15 minutes.

5. Spread the cooked beef, onion, and pine nuts over the bulgur and raw beef mixture in the baking dish. Spread the remaining raw bulgur and beef mixture on top, patting it down flat. If you're using your hands, wet them slightly to prevent the mixture from sticking. Spread the olive oil across the top. Using a sharp knife, cut the kibbeh in the pan into squares or diamonds all the way through the 3 layers.

6. Bake for 45 to 55 minutes, or until the ground beef is no longer pink and the top is browned.

7. Serve on a platter with lemon wedges and a tablespoon of Greek yogurt on each piece. Garnish with the parsley.

A single serving of this recipe is a complete 1:1:1 meal.

1:1:1 Accelerated option: Enjoy this for lunch.

10-Minute Lemon Pasta with Fresh Salmon
Serves 4

This quick-to-prepare pasta dish is a great alternative to a typical spaghetti and meatballs dinner.

> 4 (4–6 ounces each) boneless, skinless salmon fillets
> 1 tablespoon extra virgin olive oil
> Sea salt
> Freshly ground black pepper
> 12 ounces whole wheat rotini pasta
> ½ cup plain nonfat Greek yogurt
> 2 tablespoons chopped fresh basil
> 2 tablespoons freshly squeezed lemon juice
> 1 tablespoon chopped fresh rosemary
> 1 tablespoon Parmesan cheese, grated

1. Preheat the broiler. Rub the salmon fillets with the olive oil and season them with the salt and pepper. On a large baking sheet, arrange the salmon fillets. Broil until the salmon flakes easily, turning once, about 7 minutes total.

2. Meanwhile, cook the pasta according to package directions. Drain, reserving $\frac{1}{2}$ cup of the cooking liquid.

3. In a large bowl, flake the cooked salmon. Add the pasta, yogurt, basil, lemon juice, rosemary, cheese, and reserved pasta water. Stir well to mix.

A single serving of this recipe is a complete 1:1:1 meal.

1:1:1 Accelerated option: **Enjoy this for lunch.**

Whole Wheat Penne Caprese

Serves 2

This is an ideal meal for summer, when ripe tomatoes are in season.

1 pound ripe tomatoes, chopped
2 tablespoons extra virgin olive oil
1 tablespoon balsamic vinegar
1 teaspoon freshly squeezed lemon juice
$\frac{1}{2}$ teaspoon sea salt
$\frac{1}{4}$ teaspoon freshly ground black pepper
$\frac{1}{2}$ pound whole wheat penne
4 ounces fresh mozzarella cheese balls, sliced in half
$\frac{1}{4}$ cup thinly sliced fresh basil

1. In a large bowl, combine the tomatoes, olive oil, vinegar, lemon juice, salt, and pepper. Toss well and refrigerate for 1 hour.

2. Cook the pasta according to package directions until al dente. Drain and toss gently with the marinated tomato mixture. Gently toss in the cheese and basil and serve immediately.

A single serving of this recipe is a complete 1:1:1 meal.

1:1:1 Accelerated option: **Enjoy this for lunch only.**

Teriyaki Sesame Chicken

Serves 6

This savory dish is a favorite with kids. Marinating the chicken overnight infuses it with flavor.

½ cup rice wine vinegar
½ cup reduced-sodium soy sauce
½ cup water
2 tablespoons toasted sesame oil
1 tablespoon raw sugar or honey
1 clove garlic, minced
1 teaspoon grated fresh ginger
2 pounds boneless, skinless chicken breasts, cut into cubes
¼ cup sesame seeds
Cooking spray
¼ cup chopped scallions
Freshly ground black pepper

1. In a large zip-top bag, combine the vinegar, soy sauce, water, sesame oil, sugar or honey, garlic, and ginger. Add the chicken and marinate in the refrigerator for 8 hours or overnight, flipping a few times.

2. Remove the chicken and set aside. In a medium saucepan over medium-high heat, bring the marinade to a boil. Reduce the heat to low and cook until reduced slightly, about 15 minutes.

3. Meanwhile, in a dry skillet over medium heat, toast the sesame seeds, shaking the skillet occasionally until they become browned and fragrant, about 3 minutes.

4. Coat a large skillet or cast iron grill pan with cooking spray and set it over high heat. Add the chicken and cook until the meat is no longer pink, about 10 minutes. Baste the chicken with the reduced marinade. Cook for another 3 minutes.

5. Remove from the heat. Garnish with the chopped scallions and toasted sesame seeds, season with pepper, and serve.

Make it 1:1:1: Serve with a carb, such as 1 cup of jasmine or brown rice.

1:1:1 Accelerated option: For dinner, serve with sautéed vegetables such as zucchini, squash, or bok choy.

Lemon-Garlic Pesto Pasta with Kale and Asparagus

Kale and asparagus bulk up pasta without adding refined carbs or calories. Plus, they're rich in vitamins A and K. And the olive oil in this dish helps you better absorb those nutrients.

1 bunch thin asparagus, tough ends cut off
1 teaspoon + 2 tablespoons extra virgin olive oil
Salt
Freshly ground black pepper
Juice of 2 lemons
4 cloves garlic, minced
Pinch of red-pepper flakes
1 bunch kale, stemmed and chopped
12 ounces whole wheat farfalle (or other pasta shape you like)
¼ cup basil pesto (purchased or homemade with your favorite recipe)
2 pounds precooked chicken sausage, sliced

1. Preheat the oven to 350°F. On a baking sheet, arrange the asparagus in a single layer. Drizzle the asparagus with 1 teaspoon of olive oil, season it with salt and pepper, and roast for 20 to 25 minutes, or until tender.

2. Meanwhile, in a large skillet over medium heat, heat the remaining 2 tablespoons of olive oil. Add the lemon juice, garlic, and red-pepper flakes and cook until fragrant, about 2 minutes. Add the kale, cooking and stirring occasionally until wilted, about 8 minutes.

3. Meanwhile, cook the pasta according to package directions until al dente. Drain and return the pasta to the pot. Add the pesto and toss to coat. Gently toss in the asparagus, kale, and chicken sausage. Add additional salt and pepper to taste.

A single serving of this recipe is a complete 1:1:1 meal.

1:1:1 Accelerated option: **If you're having this for dinner, skip the pasta and toss the pesto with the asparagus, kale, and chicken sausage.**

Thai Chicken with Chili-Pineapple Sauce

Serves 4

Feel free to experiment and substitute shrimp or beef for the chicken or basmati or jasmine rice for basic brown or white rice.

$1\frac{1}{2}$ pounds boneless, skinless chicken thighs, cut into $\frac{1}{2}$"-wide strips

Coarse salt

Freshly ground black pepper

1 cup rice

1 tablespoon coconut oil

2 tablespoons minced garlic

1 tablespoon peeled, finely chopped fresh ginger

1 cup coconut milk (shake the can well before opening)

$1\frac{1}{2}$ cups chopped fresh pineapple, divided

2 teaspoons fish sauce

$\frac{1}{3}$ cup chopped scallions

$\frac{1}{4}$ teaspoon Thai chili paste, or to taste

1. Season the chicken with salt and pepper. Cook the rice according to package instructions.

2. In a large skillet over medium-high heat, heat the coconut oil. Cook the chicken, stirring frequently, until golden, about 10 minutes. Add the garlic and ginger and cook, stirring, until fragrant, about 1 minute. Add the coconut milk, $\frac{1}{2}$ cup of the pineapple, and the fish sauce. Bring the mixture to a light boil. Stir and reduce the heat. With the pot partially covered, simmer until the chicken is cooked through, about 10 minutes.

3. In a bowl, combine the remaining 1 cup of pineapple with the scallions and chili paste.

4. Serve the chicken over the rice, topped with the chili-pineapple sauce.

A single serving of this recipe is a complete 1:1:1 meal.

1:1:1 Accelerated option: For dinner, instead of serving this over rice, serve it over a bed of shredded cabbage or kale.

Roasted Butternut Squash and Pomegranate Salad

Hearty ingredients like rich butternut squash, chewy farro, and salty feta cheese make this salad feel indulgent, while pomegranate brightens it up.

1 butternut squash, peeled and cut into $\frac{1}{2}''$ cubes

4 tablespoons extra virgin olive oil, divided

Salt

Freshly ground black pepper

1 cup farro

1 tablespoon freshly squeezed lemon juice

1 teaspoon Dijon mustard

$\frac{1}{4}$ cup finely chopped parsley

10 cups fresh spinach

Arils from 1 pomegranate (or 1 cup arils, if purchased already removed from the fruit)

1 cup crumbled feta cheese

1. Preheat the oven to 375°F. Line a baking sheet with parchment paper.

2. Spread the butternut squash on the prepared baking sheet. Drizzle it with 2 tablespoons of the olive oil, sprinkle it with salt and pepper, and toss until evenly coated. Roast for 30 to 40 minutes, or until tender. Meanwhile, cook the farro according to package directions.

3. To make the dressing, in a small bowl, whisk together the remaining 2 tablespoons of olive oil, the lemon juice, Dijon mustard, and additional salt and pepper. Add the parsley. Set aside.

4. In a large bowl, combine the farro, spinach, and pomegranate arils. Add the butternut squash and feta cheese and stir to combine. Drizzle with the dressing.

A single serving of this recipe is a complete 1:1:1 meal.

1:1:1 Accelerated option: **For dinner, leave out the farro.**

Thai Chicken and Black Rice Salad

Serves 4

This exotic salad has a striking look because of the black rice. To julienne the fruit and vegetables, first slice them, then cut the slices into thin matchstick shapes. You can poach the chicken and make the rice ahead of time and keep them refrigerated until you're ready to make the rest of the dish. This dish is tasty served either hot or cold.

1/4 cup peanut butter

2 tablespoons honey

2 tablespoons freshly squeezed lime juice

2 teaspoons soy sauce

1 teaspoon rice wine vinegar

1 teaspoon grated fresh ginger

2 chicken breasts (about 1 pound total)

1/2 cup black or forbidden rice

5 cups butter lettuce

1 mango, peeled, pitted, and julienned

3 carrots, julienned

1 cucumber, julienned

1/2 cup fresh mint leaves

1/2 cup fresh cilantro

1. First, make the dressing. In a blender, process the peanut butter, honey, lime juice, soy sauce, vinegar, and ginger until smooth. Next, poach the chicken in salted water for 30 minutes and cook the rice according to package directions. Shred the chicken when it's finished cooking.

2. Divide the lettuce between 2 plates. Top each with half the black rice, then top the rice with the shredded chicken breast.

3. In a bowl, toss the mangos, carrots, and cucumber together. Spoon them over the chicken. Drizzle with the dressing and garnish with the mint, cilantro, and peanuts.

A single serving of this recipe is a complete 1:1:1 meal.

1:1:1 Accelerated option: **For dinner, just leave out the rice.**

Mediterranean Chicken

Serves 6

A knockout main dish, this recipe is easy to prepare. You can choose your own herbs to change the flavor. The beauty is that you can't go wrong! Cooking the chicken in the skin keeps it moist and the bone adds more flavor, but remove both before eating.

6 bone-in chicken thighs, with skin
1 tablespoon extra virgin olive oil
2 cups halved grape tomatoes
$\frac{1}{2}$ cup pitted and halved green olives or 6 ounces goat cheese, crumbled
6 medium shallots, peeled and halved
3 sprigs fresh thyme
Coarse salt
Freshly ground black pepper
Fresh mint leaves

1. Preheat the oven to 375°F. In a large bowl, combine the chicken, oil, tomatoes, olives, shallots, and thyme. Season with salt and pepper and toss.

2. In a rimmed baking sheet, spread the chicken mixture in a single layer, skin side up. Roast for 35 to 40 minutes, or until a thermometer inserted in the thickest portion of the thigh registers 170°F and the juices run clear.

3. Transfer the chicken to a platter and loosely cover it with foil. Return the vegetables to the oven and roast for another 10 minutes (or until golden brown) while the chicken is resting.

4. Spoon the vegetables and pan juices over the chicken and sprinkle with additional salt and pepper. Garnish with the mint leaves and crumbled goat cheese, if using.

Make it 1:1:1: Serve with cooked orzo.

1:1:1 Accelerated option: **No changes necessary.**

Green Curry Shrimp (or Chicken)

Serves 4

Why spend money at a restaurant when you can make this spicy and flavorful Thai dish at home for a fraction of the price (and calories!)? I love this dish, and if you're a fan of Thai food, I bet you will, too.

- **1 cup brown rice**
- **1 tablespoon peanut oil**
- **1/2 cup chopped onion**
- **2 cloves garlic, minced**
- **1 tablespoon peeled, chopped fresh ginger**
- **3–4 teaspoons green curry paste (depending how spicy you want it)**
- **3 cups fresh spinach**
- **1 cup sugar snap peas**
- **1 red bell pepper, sliced**
- **1 cup coconut milk**
- **1 pound shrimp, peeled and deveined (or 1 pound cooked, shredded chicken breast)**
- **1/4 cup chopped fresh basil**

1. Cook the rice according to package directions.

2. In a large skillet, heat the oil over medium heat. Add the onion and cook until soft, 3 to 4 minutes. Stir in the garlic, ginger, and green curry paste. Cook until fragrant, or about 30 seconds longer.

3. Add the spinach, sugar snap peas, and bell pepper slices. Cook until tender, about 5 minutes. Add the coconut milk and bring to a simmer. Add the shrimp and cook until pink, about 3 minutes. Serve over the rice, garnished with the basil.

A single serving of this recipe is a complete 1:1:1 meal.

1:1:1 Accelerated option: **Serve over shredded cabbage instead of brown rice.**

Grilled Lamb and Vegetable Skewers

Serves 4

When making skewers, thread the meat and each individual vegetable on its own skewer, so everything gets thoroughly cooked but not overdone. Skewers can be assembled up to 3 hours ahead of time, but allow them to sit at room temperature for 30 minutes before grilling.

$1\frac{1}{2}$ pounds top round lamb, cut into $1\frac{1}{2}''$ cubes
3 tablespoons extra virgin olive oil + additional for dressing
Coarse sea salt
Freshly ground black pepper
2 medium zucchini, sliced 1" thick
16 medium cipollini or pearl onions, peeled (or 1 large onion cut into 2" wedges)
16 medium button or baby bella mushrooms, trimmed
Zest and juice of 1 lemon
$\frac{1}{2}$ cup coarsely chopped fresh flat-leaf parsley

1. Preheat the grill to medium-high heat. Soak twelve 12" wooden skewers in water for 30 minutes, then drain.

2. In a bowl, toss the lamb with 1 tablespoon of oil and sprinkle it with salt and pepper.

3. In a different bowl, toss the zucchini, onions, and mushrooms with 2 tablespoons of oil and season with additional salt and pepper.

4. Divide the lamb among 4 skewers and thread the zucchini, onions, and mushrooms on separate skewers.

5. Place the lamb and mushroom skewers on the grill and cook for 10 minutes. Add the zucchini skewers and cook for 8 minutes. Add the onion skewers and cook for 5 minutes. Remember to turn all the skewers occasionally.

6. Remove all skewers from the grill and dress them with the lemon zest and juice, a bit of olive oil, and the parsley. Each person can get one of each kind.

Make it 1:1:1: Serve alongside a carb, such as rice, couscous, or potato salad.

1:1:1 Accelerated option: No changes necessary, but add a green salad if you like.

Chicken Tortilla Soup

Serves 6

Chicken tortilla soup is comfort food, and so easy to make that you could have it every week! To save even more time, crumble store-bought baked tortilla chips on top instead of making your own.

3 tablespoons peanut oil, divided
1 small onion, finely chopped
2 cloves garlic, minced
6 cups low-sodium chicken broth
1 can (15 ounces) diced tomatoes, with liquid
1 tablespoon tomato paste
1 tablespoon + 1 teaspoon chili powder
Coarse salt
Freshly ground black pepper
3 boneless, skinless chicken breasts, cut into bite-sized cubes (3 pounds total)
3 corn tortillas, cut into thin strips
1 avocado, thinly sliced, or 1 cup (2 ounces) crumbled Cotija cheese
$\frac{1}{4}$ cup fresh cilantro leaves
1 scallion, thinly sliced
1 lime, cut into 6 wedges

1. Preheat the oven to 400°F.

2. In a large pot, heat 1 tablespoon of the oil over medium-high heat. Cook the onions until almost translucent, or about 3 to 4 minutes. Add the garlic and cook until fragrant, about another 30 seconds. Add the chicken broth, tomatoes and liquid, tomato paste, and chili powder. Season with the salt and pepper. Bring the mixture to a boil.

3. Lower the heat to simmer, and add the chicken. Simmer until the chicken is cooked through, 15 to 20 minutes. Taste and add more salt and pepper, if necessary.

4. On a baking sheet, toss the tortilla strips with 2 tablespoons of the oil. Bake until crisp and golden brown, tossing halfway through, or for a total of 15 to 20 minutes.

5. To serve, divide the soup among 6 bowls and garnish with the tortilla strips, avocado or cheese, cilantro, and scallion. Serve with the lime wedges.

This a complete 1:1:1 meal as is.

1:1:1 Accelerated option: **Just skip the tortilla strips and you're good to go!**

Salmon Cakes on Mixed Greens

Serves 4

This healthful but elegant meal is easier than it looks, and a more nutritious choice than burgers.

$1\frac{1}{2}$ pounds boneless, skinless salmon fillets

1 cup panko bread crumbs

$\frac{1}{4}$ cup mayonnaise

2 eggs, lightly beaten

2 tablespoons capers

3 tablespoons finely chopped fresh dill, divided

2 tablespoons finely chopped onion

1 tablespoon Dijon mustard

1 teaspoon Old Bay seasoning

Sea salt

Freshly ground black pepper

8 tablespoons extra virgin olive oil, divided

$\frac{1}{4}$ cup rice wine vinegar

$1\frac{1}{2}$ tablespoons freshly squeezed lemon juice

1 tablespoon coarse-grain mustard

12 cups mixed greens or spring greens

$\frac{1}{4}$ cup chopped flat-leaf parsley

1. Preheat the oven to 400°F. Place the salmon fillets on a baking sheet covered in parchment paper and roast for 15 minutes. Flake the cooked salmon in a medium mixing bowl. Reduce the oven temperature to 375°F.

2. In the same mixing bowl, place the bread crumbs, mayonnaise, eggs, capers, 2 tablespoons of the fresh dill, onion, Dijon mustard, Old Bay seasoning, salt, and pepper. Stir gently until combined well with the salmon.

3. Using your hands, form the mixture into 8 disk-shaped cakes.

4. In an ovenproof skillet over medium-high heat, heat 4 tablespoons of the oil. Cook the salmon cakes until browned, about 2 minutes on each side. Transfer the skillet to the oven and bake for an additional 8 minutes.

5. In a large bowl, whisk together the remaining 4 tablespoons of oil, the vinegar, lemon juice, remaining 1 tablespoon of dill, coarse-grain mustard, and additional pepper. Toss the mixed greens with the dressing.

6. Divide the salad greens evenly among 4 plates and top each with 2 salmon cakes. Season with additional pepper and garnish with the parsley.

This a complete 1:1:1 meal.

1:1:1 Accelerated option: **Reserve this meal for lunch—the bread crumbs make it inappropriate for an Accelerated dinner.**

Chicken Sumac

Serves 8

Using bone-in chicken and leaving the skin on adds more flavor to the finished dish. You can also increase the flavor by using a good-quality olive oil and covering the chicken for 10 to 15 minutes after you dress it. If you have leftovers, make a wrap for lunch the next day.

3 pounds bone-in chicken pieces, with skin
$\frac{1}{4}$ cup extra virgin olive oil
Salt
Freshly ground black pepper
$2\frac{1}{2}$ cups chopped red onions
$\frac{1}{4}$ cup ground sumac (available at many specialty stores)
$\frac{1}{2}$ cup toasted pine nuts

1. Preheat the oven to 400°F. Place the chicken in a 13″ x 9″ baking pan, brush it with 1 tablespoon olive oil, and sprinkle it with salt and pepper.

2. Bake for about 45 minutes, or until a thermometer inserted in the thickest portion registers 170°F and the juices run clear.

3. While the chicken is baking, in a medium saucepan, cook the red onions in 1 tablespoon of the olive oil until soft, about 10 minutes. Set aside.

4. When the chicken is cooked, allow to cool, then remove the skin and bones. Shred the meat and place it in a bowl.

5. In a separate bowl, combine the remaining 2 tablespoons olive oil, sumac, and salt to taste.

6. Dress the shredded chicken with the olive oil mixture.

7. Top the chicken with the onions and pine nuts. Use clean hands to mix all ingredients thoroughly.

To make a wrap:

1. Preheat the oven to 350°F. Place ¾ cup Chicken Sumac in a whole wheat, high-fiber, or white flour tortilla and fold it like a burrito.

2. Lightly brush the wrap with olive oil and bake it for 5 to 7 minutes, or until golden.

3. Cut in half and enjoy.

Make it 1:1:1: In a wrap, a single serving of Chicken Sumac is a complete 1:1:1 meal. Instead of a tortilla, you could also have rice as your carb.

1:1:1 Accelerated option: Enjoy this with a dollop of plain low-fat or whole-fat yogurt and a side salad.

Side Dishes

These delicious sides can be a part of any meal. For each, I highlight which micronutrients the recipe contains, and you make it a complete meal or pair it with its missing element any way you choose.

18-Carrot-Gold Salad

Serves 4

This quick, easy variation on potato salad has an exotic twist and is extremely satisfying. This recipe has a carb and a fat.

2 cups diced (½″) red potatoes
Sea salt
Freshly ground black pepper
1 cup shredded carrots
1 cup shredded cabbage
½ cup walnuts
½ cup yellow curry sauce*
⅓ cup golden raisins
⅓ cup low-fat mayonnaise

1. In a medium saucepan, cover the potatoes with water. Bring to a boil, then simmer until tender, about 15 minutes. Drain, then season with salt and pepper and set aside to cool.

2. In a large bowl, mix together the potatoes, carrots, cabbage, walnuts, curry sauce, raisins, and mayonnaise. Chill in the refrigerator for at least 2 hours. Serve cold.

*If you can't find bottled curry sauce, you can make your own by adding 2 tablespoons of curry powder to $\frac{1}{2}$ cup of low-fat mayonnaise.

Three-Bean Salad

Serves 4

You can mix and match the types of beans you use in this salad to include your favorites. It's so simple and fresh! This recipe has a fat and either a carb or protein in the beans.

$\frac{3}{4}$ **cup canned chickpeas, rinsed and drained**
$\frac{3}{4}$ **cup canned kidney beans, rinsed and drained**
$\frac{3}{4}$ **cup canned black beans, rinsed and drained**
$\frac{1}{2}$ **cup chopped cucumbers**
$\frac{1}{2}$ **cup chopped tomatoes**
2 tablespoons kalamata olives
2 tablespoons extra virgin olive oil
2 tablespoons white wine vinegar
1 tablespoon freshly squeezed lemon juice
Salt
Freshly ground black pepper

1. In a mixing bowl, combine the chickpeas, kidney beans, black beans, cucumbers, tomatoes, and olives.

2. Dress with the oil, vinegar, and lemon juice. Stir to evenly distribute the dressing, add the salt and pepper to taste, and serve.

Curried Corn Slaw

Serves 8

An exotic twist on a classic, this colorful side dish is full of fiber, anti-oxidants, and flavor. It pairs nicely with meat or beans. This recipe is a carb and a fat.

3 cups shredded cabbage
2 cups chopped broccoli
2 cups shredded carrots
1 ear sweet corn (or $\frac{1}{2}$ cup frozen corn)
$\frac{1}{4}$ cup low-fat mayonnaise
$\frac{1}{4}$ cup yellow curry sauce*
$\frac{1}{4}$ cup golden raisins

1. In a large bowl, combine the cabbage, broccoli, and carrots. Shave the sweet corn kernels into the bowl.

2. In a medium bowl, combine the mayonnaise and yellow curry sauce. Dress the salad with the sauce, sprinkle in the raisins, and stir to combine.

*If you can't find bottled curry sauce, you can make your own by adding 2 tablespoons of curry powder to $\frac{1}{2}$ cup of low-fat mayonnaise.

Serve-It-on-the-Side Salad

Use whatever quantity of vegetables you prefer to create your own salad masterpiece! This recipe is "free"!

Tomatoes
Persian cucumbers
Jalapeño chile peppers, seeded (wear plastic gloves when handling)
Scallions (optional)
Equal parts extra virgin olive oil, white wine vinegar, and freshly squeezed lemon juice
Salt
Freshly ground black pepper
Chopped cilantro

1. Chop the tomatoes, cucumbers, jalapeño peppers, and scallions.

2. In a bowl, combine the chopped vegetables. Dress with the oil, vinegar, and lemon juice. Toss until well combined. Add salt and black pepper to taste, top with the cilantro, and serve.

Super-Antioxidant Beet Salad

This high-potency salad is rich in antioxidants and big on taste. You could also add mixed greens if you desire. This recipe is a carb and a fat

6 cups cooked beets, cut into small cubes
1 cup pomegranate arils (optional)
$3/4$ cup dried cranberries
$1/2$ cup chopped walnuts
Raspberry vinaigrette

1. In a large bowl, combine the beets, pomegranate arils (if using), cranberries, and walnuts.

2. Add the raspberry vinaigrette to taste, and toss.

Lady Green with Envy

Serves 6

A high-fiber mix of lightly stir-fried, heart-healthy green veggies! This recipe is "free"!

1 tablespoon extra virgin olive oil
2 cups broccoli florets
2 cups asparagus
2 cups chopped (1") sugar snap peas
½ cup teriyaki sauce

In a large skillet, over medium-high heat, heat the olive oil. Sauté the broccoli, asparagus, and sugar snap peas, stirring frequently, until tender but crisp and bright green, about 4 minutes. Add the teriyaki sauce and toss. Remove from the heat and serve.

Artichoke Salad

Serves 1

A flavor-full Italian-style salad, this dish is great year-round. You can also add seasonal veggies to bump up the fiber content. This recipe is a fat.

1 cup baby spinach
¼ cup marinated artichoke hearts
¼ cup halved grape tomatoes
2 tablespoons kalamata olives
1 tablespoon chopped red onions
1 tablespoon shaved Parmigiano–Reggiano cheese
2 teaspoons extra virgin olive oil
1 teaspoon balsamic vinegar

Place the spinach on a plate. Top it with the artichoke hearts, then the tomatoes, the olives, the onions, and the cheese. Drizzle with the oil and vinegar.

Tabbouleh Salad

Tabbouleh is a staple in the Mediterranean diet and I eat it frequently. It's chewy, filling, and satisfying, as well as nutritionally dense, so the nutritionist in me gives this a gold star! This recipe is a carb and a fat.

- ½ cup fine-grade bulgur
- 5 bunches (3 cups) parsley (flat leaf or curly, whichever you prefer)
- 2 tablespoons finely chopped fresh mint
- 4 scallions, finely chopped
- 6 medium tomatoes, finely chopped
- A few leaves romaine lettuce
- ¼ cup + 2 tablespoons extra virgin olive oil
- ¼ cup + 2 tablespoons freshly squeezed lemon juice
- 1 tablespoon salt
- ½ teaspoon freshly ground black pepper

1. In a bowl, soak the bulgur in enough boiling water to just cover it for 1 hour, or until soft and fluffy. Squeeze the excess water from the bulgur using your hands or a paper towel.

2. Separate the parsley leaves from the stems. Wash the leaves thoroughly in a colander and lay them on a paper towel or dish towel to dry completely. Then finely chop them.

3. In a medium bowl, combine the bulgur, parsley, mint, scallions, and tomatoes. Line a serving bowl with the lettuce and transfer the bulgur mixture to that bowl.

4. Sprinkle the oil, lemon juice, salt, and pepper on top of the bulgur mixture. Serve immediately or chill in the refrigerator for up to 2 hours. Before you serve this dish, make sure to stir it from the bottom to the top to ensure that you get all of the flavor from the oil and lemon juice.

Summer Slaw

Serves 4

This light salad is a great addition to any summer dinner. Bursting with vibrant colors from apples, red cabbage, carrots, and chard, this slaw also bursts with nutrients. This is a healthy and light side dish that will also squash any late-night cravings. This recipe is a carb.

  2 apples, cubed
  1 cup grated red cabbage
  1 cup grated carrots
  1 cup thinly sliced chard leaves
  ½ cup chopped fresh flat-leaf parsley
  2 tablespoons apple cider vinegar
  2 tablespoons freshly squeezed lemon juice
  2 tablespoons extra virgin olive oil
  1 teaspoon honey
  Sea salt
  Freshly ground black pepper

In a large bowl, combine the apples, cabbage, carrots, chard, parsley, vinegar, lemon juice, oil, honey, and salt and pepper to taste. Toss well to coat. Serve immediately or let sit overnight to allow the flavors to develop.

Beet-Infused Ruby Quinoa

Serves 2

This tasty and vibrant dish is a carb and a protein recipe.

  ½ cup quinoa, washed and drained
  1 cup water
  1 cup grated fresh beets, washed and peeled
  2 tablespoons chopped fresh chives
  1 tablespoon extra virgin olive oil
  1 teaspoon grated lemon zest
  Sea salt
  Freshly ground black pepper

1. In a medium pot over high heat, bring the quinoa and water to a boil. Cover and simmer gently until the liquid is absorbed, about 10 minutes. (Do not overcook, or the quinoa will become mushy.)

2. Remove from the heat. Add the beets, chives, oil, lemon zest, and salt and pepper to taste. Stir until the ruby color from the beets is evenly distributed. Cover and allow to cool for 10 minutes before serving.

Vanilla-Orange Mashed Sweet Potatoes

Serves 4

This recipe is great as a side dish, but with its natural sugars and caramelization, it works just as well as a healthy dessert. This recipe is a carb and a fat.

3 pounds sweet potatoes
$\frac{1}{2}$ cup light, unsweetened canned coconut milk
1 tablespoon honey
1 teaspoon orange zest
1 teaspoon vanilla extract
$\frac{1}{4}$ teaspoon ground cinnamon
Pinch of sea salt

1. Preheat the oven to 450°F. On a foil-lined baking sheet, roast the sweet potatoes for 1 hour or until very soft, turning once. Remove from the oven and cool slightly.

2. When cool enough to handle, scoop the flesh into a large bowl and discard the skins. Add the coconut milk, honey, orange zest, vanilla, cinnamon, and salt and mash well. Serve warm.

Green Papaya Salad

Serves 8

This unusual salad is inspired by a traditional Thai dish, but I've mixed it with some salad greens for more fiber and nutrition. Many Asian supermarkets sell shredded green papaya, but if you can't find it, try making this with 4 large green apples, cored and chopped. Or, for a twist, try about 3 cups of chopped English (seedless) cucumber. It will be much different, but it will still be delicious. This recipe is a fat.

- ⅓ cup honey
- ⅓ cup unseasoned rice wine vinegar
- ¼ cup soy sauce
- ¼ cup toasted sesame oil
- ¼ cup extra virgin olive oil
- 1 teaspoon Sriracha (or any hot sauce)
- 8 cups salad greens, torn into bite-sized pieces
- 1 green papaya, peeled, halved, seeded, and julienned
- 1 cup torn fresh Thai basil leaves
- ½ cup cilantro leaves or flat-leaf parsley
- ½ cup sliced almonds

1. In a small bowl, whisk together the honey, vinegar, soy sauce, sesame oil, olive oil, and Sriracha. Set aside.

2. In a large bowl, combine the salad greens, papaya, basil, and cilantro. Drizzle with the dressing and toss to coat everything. Serve topped with the sliced almonds.

Marinated Summer Vegetables

Serves 8

This dish can be made up to 3 days ahead of time but should be brought to room temperature before serving. This recipe is a carb.

- 3 zucchini, diagonally sliced into ½"-thick slices
- 3 bell peppers, cut into 1" strips
- 4 tablespoons extra-virgin olive oil, divided
- Coarse salt
- Freshly ground black pepper
- 2 cloves garlic, minced
- 2 tablespoons red wine vinegar
- 3 cups corn kernals, cooked
- 4 sprigs rosemary

1. Place racks in the upper and lower thirds of the oven and preheat it to 475°F.

2. On 2 separate baking sheets, place the zucchini and bell peppers. Drizzle each sheet of vegetables with ½ tablespoon of the oil, season with salt and pepper, and toss to coat. Spread out the vegetables in a single layer, turning the peppers skin side up.

3. Roast the peppers on the upper rack and the zucchini on the lower rack for 15 to 20 minutes or until tender, turning the zucchini once. Let cool slightly, then remove the skins from the peppers.

4. In a large bowl, whisk the garlic, vinegar, and remaining 3 tablespoons of oil. Season with additional salt and pepper. Add the zucchini, bell peppers, corn, and rosemary and toss to coat. Cover and let sit for at least 1 hour.

Spicy Baby Bok Choy

Serves 4

This spicy Asian side dish pairs well with any fish, shrimp, or even grilled steak. This recipe is a fat.

¼ cup peanut oil
1 piece (½") fresh ginger, peeled and finely chopped
2 cloves garlic, minced
8 baby bok choy, halved lengthwise
¼ cup water
Juice of 1 lemon
½ teaspoon sea salt
Pinch of hot-pepper flakes

1. In a large skillet over medium-high heat, heat the oil. Stir in the ginger and garlic and cook until fragrant, about 30 seconds.

2. Add the bok choy and water and immediately cover the skillet. Cook, turning the bok choy once, until bok choy is tender, about 3 minutes.

3. Uncover the skillet and add the lemon juice, salt, and hot-pepper flakes. Stir for 1 minute, then serve hot.

Indian-Style Cauliflower

Serves 8

Look for whole spices in your natural foods store or ethnic grocery store. This recipe is "free"!

2 tablespoons extra virgin olive oil
1 teaspoon coriander seeds
1 teaspoon cumin seeds
1 teaspoon curry powder
1 teaspoon ground turmeric
1 large head cauliflower, cored and broken into 1" florets
Sea salt
Freshly ground black pepper
1 teaspoon finely grated fresh ginger
1 teaspoon finely grated lime zest

1. Preheat the oven to 450°F. In a large bowl, whisk together the oil, coriander seeds, cumin seeds, curry, and turmeric. Add the cauliflower and season with salt and pepper. Toss until coated evenly.

2. On a large rimmed baking sheet, arrange the cauliflower in a single layer (scrape any extra seasoning from the bowl over the cauliflower). Roast until the cauliflower is brown around the edges and crisp-tender, 10 to 15 minutes.

3. Transfer to a platter and sprinkle with the ginger and lime zest. Serve warm or at room temperature.

Snacks

Sweet or savory, snacks keep you going. Here are some of my favorites. Most of them are balanced for 1:1:1 (I let you know when you need to add something). All are acceptable if you are on 1:1:1 Accelerated.

Coconut-Honey Carrots

Serves 2

This deliciously simple dish feels exotic and special.

1 cup baby carrots
2 tablespoons coconut
1 tablespoon honey

1. Bring a pot of water to a boil. Boil the carrots until tender, about 10 minutes, and then drain. Meanwhile, in a skillet over medium heat, toast the coconut by stirring frequently until mostly golden brown.

2. Place the carrots on a plate and drizzle them with the honey.

3. Sprinkle the toasted coconut on top.

Make it 1:1:1: Enjoy with $\frac{1}{2}$ cup of ricotta or a dollop of crème fraiche to make it 1:1:1.

Zucchini Chip Muffins

Serves 12

My clients know that I love dark chocolate chips! Using them in baked goods allows you to have a treat that will satisfy your cravings without going overboard. These muffins have been enhanced with shredded zucchini to keep them moist, which also adds fiber and allows you to use less flour.

Cooking spray
1½ cups fat-free milk
¾ cup plain nonfat yogurt
½ cup sugar
1 cup unsweetened applesauce or mashed banana
2 cups whole wheat pastry flour
3 tablespoons unsweetened cocoa powder
2 teaspoons ground cinnamon
1¼ teaspoons baking soda
¼ teaspoon salt
1½ cups finely shredded zucchini
½ cup semisweet dark chocolate chips

1. Preheat the oven to 350°F and generously spray a 12-cup, standard-sized muffin tin with cooking spray.

2. In a large bowl, combine the milk, yogurt, and sugar. Mix well until creamy. Stir in the applesauce or banana and mix well again.

3. In a separate bowl, combine the flour, cocoa, cinnamon, baking soda, and salt. Add the dry mixture to the wet ingredients, stirring until just combined. Fold in the zucchini and chocolate chips until well incorporated.

4. Divide the batter evenly among the muffin cups. Bake for 20 minutes, or until a toothpick inserted in the center of a muffin comes out clean. Cool for at least 20 minutes before serving.

Make it 1:1:1: Top with a 1 tablespoon butter and pair with protein, such as milk or Greek yogurt.

Graham Dippers

Unlike other graham crackers you may have in your pantry, Erewhon Organic Grahams are made with all organic ingredients, plus they contain no trans fat. I like to use the honey flavor for this fun and sweet snack. The ricotta cheese adds 7 grams of muscle-building protein, and the cinnamon helps maintain steady blood sugar levels.

Sprinkle of ground cinnamon
$\frac{1}{4}$ cup low-fat ricotta cheese
1 serving Honey Graham Crackers
1 teaspoon chopped peanuts or almonds

In a small bowl, stir the cinnamon into the ricotta. Use it as a spread for the crackers and top with chopped nuts.

Fresh Figs and Cherries with Honey-Lemon Goat Cheese

This recipe is versatile—you can enjoy it as a light breakfast, a mid-morning snack, an appetizer, or even a dessert. A Mediterranean dish, it's nutrient rich and high in protein, calcium, and antioxidants.

12 figs
$\frac{1}{2}$ cup halved and pitted cherries
$\frac{1}{4}$ cup crumbled goat cheese
5 fresh basil leaves, cut into strips
1 tablespoon extra virgin olive oil
1 tablespoon freshly squeezed lemon juice
1 teaspoon honey
$\frac{1}{4}$ teaspoon sea salt

1. Slice each fig as though you are going to quarter it, but don't cut all the way to the bottom. Leave the bottoms intact, and gently pull each quarter outward, forming fig "flowers."

2. Place the figs on a serving platter and scatter the cherries around the figs.

3. Top each fig with a bit of cheese, and scatter extra cheese around the cherries on the serving platter. Sprinkle with the basil.

4. In a small bowl, whisk together the oil, lemon juice, honey, and salt.

5. With a small spoon, lightly drizzle the sauce over the entire platter. Serve immediately.

Cocoa Bananas

Serves 2

These banana slices taste almost like candy!

> 2 tablespoons unsweetened coconut
> 2 tablespoons unsweetened cocoa powder
> Pinch of salt
> Pinch of ground cinnamon (optional)
> 2 medium bananas, sliced
> $\frac{1}{2}$ cup Greek yogurt

1. In a skillet, toast the coconut by stirring it frequently over medium heat until mostly golden brown. Remove from the heat.

2. In a large zip-top bag or a bowl with a tight-fitting lid, place the coconut, cocoa powder, salt, and cinnamon (if using). Shake until well combined. Add the banana slices. Shake to coat. Pour the bananas into 2 bowls and top with the Greek yogurt.

Open-Faced Tea Sandwiches

Serves 4

So dainty, so delicious! This recipe can serve as a light lunch if you double the amount (or use this recipe to serve 2 people instead of 4) and add a mixed green salad.

    2 tablespoons crème fraiche or Greek yogurt
    1 teaspoon freshly squeezed lemon juice
    $\frac{1}{8}$ teaspoon freshly ground black pepper
    8 rye crisps or 16 rice crackers
    1 avocado, thinly sliced
    4 ounces thinly sliced smoked salmon
    16 thin slices English (seedless) cucumber

1. In a small bowl, combine the crème fraiche or yogurt, lemon juice, and pepper.

2. Spread each rye crisp or cracker with the crème fraiche mixture. Top with the avocado, smoked salmon, and cucumber slices.

Apricot-Cheese Canapés

Serves 2

This seems like a fancy hors d'oeuvre, but it's actually quite simple to make and an interesting combination of sweet and savory.

    16 dried apricots
    8 teaspoons crumbled goat cheese
    2 ounces unsalted pistachios, shelled and chopped
    $\frac{1}{2}$ teaspoon honey
    Freshly ground black pepper

On a platter, arrange the apricots. Top each apricot with $\frac{1}{2}$ teaspoon of the cheese. Then evenly top the cheese with the pistachios, a drizzle of the honey, and the pepper.

Cottage Cheese Dip with Vegetables

Serves 1

This recipe couldn't be easier or faster. Just use the cottage cheese as a dip!

$\frac{1}{2}$ cup low-fat cottage cheese
$\frac{1}{4}$ teaspoon freshly ground black pepper
$\frac{1}{2}$ cup baby carrots
$\frac{1}{2}$ cup broccoli florets
$\frac{1}{2}$ cup sliced cucumber
$\frac{1}{2}$ cup chopped (1") ribs celery

In a bowl, combine the cottage cheese and pepper. Serve with the carrots, broccoli, cucumber, and celery.

Make it 1:1:1: Serve with whole grain crackers or pita chips.

Indian-Spiced Crunchy Chickpeas

Serves 4

If you've never roasted chickpeas before, you have to try them—they're amazing! You can make this delicious snack up to 2 days in advance. Store it at room temperature.

1 can (15 ounces) chickpeas, drained and rinsed
1 tablespoon extra virgin olive oil
2 teaspoons ground cumin
1 teaspoon dried marjoram
$\frac{1}{4}$ teaspoon ground allspice
$\frac{1}{4}$ teaspoon salt

1. Position a rack in the upper third of the oven and preheat the oven to 450°F. Blot the chickpeas dry. In a bowl, toss the chickpeas with the oil, cumin, marjoram, allspice, and salt. Spread on a rimmed baking sheet.

2. Bake, stirring once or twice, for 25 to 30 minutes, until browned and crunchy. Let cool on the baking sheet for 15 minutes—if you can wait that long!

Make it 1:1:1: Pair this with a protein or a carb (chickpeas can be either one). Try dried apricots for a carb, or a chicken skewer or any leftover meat (3 ounces) for a protein addition.

Afternoon Antipasto

Serves 1

1 slice whole wheat bread, cubed
10 cherry tomatoes, halved or quartered
1 ounce mozzarella cheese, cubed
6 oil-cured olives, pitted

In a bowl, stir together the bread, tomatoes, cheese, and olives. Serve on a plate or put in a portable container and take it to-go!

Apple-Cheese Turkey Wraps

Serves 1

1 ounce any cheese, cut into strips
½ green apple, cut into thin strips
3 ounces deli turkey (about 3 slices)

Roll the cheese and apple strips inside each turkey slice.

Spicy Mango Slices

Serves 4

The unusual combination of flavors in this snack will keep your taste-buds happy until your next meal.

> **1 mango, pitted, peeled, and cut into strips**
> **Juice of 1 lime**
> **¼ cup goat cheese**
> **¼ teaspoon chili powder**

In a bowl, toss the mango slices with the lime juice. Arrange on a platter or large plate. Spread the cheese on each mango slice and sprinkle with the chili powder.

Make it 1:1:1: Adding almonds makes this a complete 1:1:1 snack.

Strawberry-Balsamic Parfait

Serves 1

> **½ cup nonfat Greek yogurt**
> **½ cup sliced strawberries**
> **1 tablespoon balsamic vinegar**
> **10 hazelnuts, chopped**
> **2 fresh mint leaves, cut into strips**

Put the yogurt in a bowl and top it with the strawberries. Drizzle with the vinegar and sprinkle with the nuts and mint.

Baked Sweet Potato Chips

Serves 2

Potato chips—but better! Sweet potatoes are rich in antioxidants and fiber.

   1 sweet potato, peeled and thinly sliced
   2 tablespoons extra virgin olive oil
   Fine sea salt
   Freshly ground black pepper
   Paprika

1. Preheat the oven to 400°F.

2. Brush both sides of the sweet potato slices with the oil and place the slices on a nonstick baking sheet.

3. Sprinkle to taste with the salt, pepper, and paprika.

4. Bake for 15 minutes. Cool on a rack.

Make it 1:1:1: Mix ½ cup Greek yogurt with 1 teaspoon curry powder and use it as a dip.

Grown-Up Ants on a Log

Serves 1

Like the kids' version, but so much better—and it's Accelerated, if you let the almond butter serve as both your protein and your fat. The cranberries are your carb.

   1 tablespoon almond butter
   2 ribs celery, leaves removed
   ¼ cup dried cranberries
   Pinch of ground cinnamon

Spread the almond butter on the celery ribs. Sprinkle each with the cranberries and cinnamon.

Make it 1:1:1: Serve with 1 cup of milk.

Index

Underscored page references indicate boxed text.

A

Abdominal fat, 180
Accelerated 1:1:1 program
  double-doers in, 118–19
  eating out on, 153, 155–64
  exercise and, 173
  food diary examples, 124–27
  meal planning for, 116–22, 142
  mixed foods in, 144
  overview, 109–11, 114–16
  vs. regular program, 112–13, 145
Acid reflux, 73–74
Adrenaline, 180
Aerobics, 171
After-dinner snacks, 53–54, 73, 136
Aging, 188
Alcoholic beverages, 64, 65, 111, 145,
  153, 157
Almonds/almond butter
  Almond-Berry Muesli, 198
  Grown-Up Ants on a Log, 260
  Mixed Berry French Toast Bake, 208
  as snack, 55
American cuisine restaurant dining
  tips, 154–55
Amino acids, 48, 51
Animal products, 23–26
Antioxidants, 162
Anxiety, 186
Appetite
  blood sugar effects, 43
  controlling, tips for, 48–49, 134–35
  excess hunger, 135, 151, 152
  exercise and, 167
  leptin and, 54
Appetizers, in restaurants, 152–53
Apples
  Almond-Berry Muesli, 198
  Apple-Cheese Turkey Wraps, 258
  Green Papaya Salad, 248–49
  Summer Slaw, 247

Apricots
  Apricot-Cheese Canapés, 256
Artichokes
  Artichoke Salad, 245
  Mediterranean Omelet, 204
Artificial sweeteners, 34, 118
Arugula
  Mediterranean Quinoa Bowl,
    213–14
  portion sizes, 67
Asian-style cuisine
  recipes
    Butternut Squash Curry,
      216–17
    Curried Corn Slaw, 243
    Green Curry Shrimp (or
      Chicken), 235
    Green Papaya Salad, 248–49
    Spicy Bok Choy, 250
    Teriyaki Sesame Chicken,
      229–30
    Thai Chicken and Black Rice
      Salad, 233
    Thai Chicken Noodle Dinner,
      223–24
    Thai Chicken with Chili-
      Pineapple Sauce, 231
    Thai-Inspired Fish en Papillote,
      214–15
  restaurant dining tips, 156–58
Asparagus
  as free food, 67
  Lady Green with Envy, 245
  Lemon-Garlic Pesto Pasta with Kale
    and Asparagus, 230
  Summer Farmers' Market Frittata,
    197–98
Avocados
  ABC Tacos, 215–16
  as fat, 142
  Open-Faced Tea Sandwiches, 256
  portion sizes, 66